Interpreting
Difficult ECGs
A RAPID REFERENCE

R

Interpreting Difficult ECGs

A RAPID REFERENCE

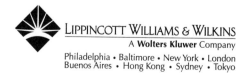

LIPPINCOTT WILLIAMS & WILKINS
A **Wolters Kluwer** Company

Philadelphia • Baltimore • New York • London
Buenos Aires • Hong Kong • Sydney • Tokyo

STAFF

Executive Publisher
Judith A. Schilling McCann,
RN,MSN

Editorial Director
H. Nancy Holmes

Clinical Director
Joan M. Robinson, RN, MSN

Senior Art Director
Arlene Putterman

Editorial Project Manager
Jennifer Lynn Kowalak

Clinical Project Manager
Mary Perrong, RN, CRNP, MSN,
APRN,BC

Editors
Stacey A. Follin, Julie Munden

Clinical Editor
Kate McGovern, RN, MSN, CCRN

Copy Editors
Kimberly Bilotta (supervisor),
Tom DeZego, Jen Fielding,
Danielle Michaely,
Kelly Pavlovsky,
Pamela Wingrod

**Digital Composition
Services**
Diane Paluba (manager),
Donna S. Morris (project
manager), Joyce Rossi Biletz

Manufacturing
Patricia K. Dorshaw (director),
Beth J. Welsh

Editorial Assistants
Megan L. Aldinger, Karen J. Kirk,
Linda K. Ruhf

Design Assistant
Georg Purvis, 4th

Indexer
Barbara Hodgson

The clinical treatments described and recommended in this publication are based on research and consultation with nursing, medical, and legal authorities. To the best of our knowledge, these procedures reflect currently accepted practice. Nevertheless, they can't be considered absolute and universal recommendations. For individual applications, all recommendations must be considered in light of the patient's clinical condition and, before administration of new or infrequently used drugs, in light of the latest package-insert information. The authors and publisher disclaim any responsibility for any adverse effects resulting from the suggested procedures, from any undetected errors, or from the reader's misunderstanding of the text.

DIFFECGS011205 — D
07 06 05   10 9 8 7 6 5 4 3 2 1

**Library of Congress
Cataloging-in-Publication Data**
Interpreting difficult ECGs : a rapid reference.
    p. ; cm.
  Includes bibliographical references and index.
  1. Electrocardiography — Interpretation. 2.
Heart — Diseases — Diagnosis. 3. Heart —
Diseases — Treatment.
  [DNLM: 1. Electrocardiography — methods. 2.
Heart Diseases — diagnosis. 3. Heart Diseases —
therapy. WG 140 I6196 2006] I. Lippincott Williams
& Wilkins.
RC683.5.E5I58 2006
616.1'207547 — dc22
  ISBN 1-58255-447-1 (alk. paper)   2005026308

Contents

Contributors and consultants

Natalie Burkhalter, RN, MSN, FNP-BC, ACNP-BC, CCRN
Associate Professor
Texas A&M International University
Laredo

Marissa Camanga-Reyes, RN, MN, CNS, CCRN
Nurse-Manager
Harbor–University of California at Los Angeles Medical Center
Torrance

Sara L. Clutter, RN, MSN
Assistant Professor of Nursing
Waynesburg (Pa.) College

Leslie Louise Davis, RN, MSN, CS, ANP
Clinical Associate Professor
University of North Carolina
Chapel Hill

Sandra Hamilton, RN, BSN, MEd, CRNI
Nurse Liaison
Resource Pharmacy
Henderson, Nev.

Timothy Hudson, RN, BSN, MS, MEd, CCRN, CHE, CNA
Nurse-Manager, ICU
Womack U.S. Army Medical Center
Fort Bragg, N.C.

Manon Lemonde, RN, PhD
Associate Professor
Faculty of Health Sciences
University of Ontario Institute of Technology
Oshawa

Amy Shay, RN, MS, CCRN, CNS
Pulmonary CNS
Miami Valley Hospital
Dayton, Ohio

Alexander John Siomko, RN,BC, MSN, CRNP, APRN,BC
Staff Nurse
Methodist Hospital Division
Thomas Jefferson University Hospital
Philadelphia

Rita M. Wick, RN, BSN
Education Specialist
Berkshire Health Systems
Pittsfield, Mass.

Shu-Fen Wung, RN, PhD, ACNP,BC, FAHA
Associate Professor
University of Arizona
Tucson

Foreword

I've been teaching interpretation of electrocardiograms (ECGs) and rhythm strips to nurses, nursing students, and advanced practice nurses for almost three decades and one of the greatest challenges is always selecting the textbook — what's the *best* ECG book to have in the personal library? The resounding answer is *Interpreting Difficult ECGs: A Rapid Reference*. This book begins with a comprehensive overview of the cardiovascular system, including cardiac anatomy and physiology, and then proceeds directly to techniques for reading ECGs. Indeed, the 8-step process is the focal point of the text. There's also a unique and useful chapter on bedside ECG monitoring systems and troubleshooting monitor problems.

The core of the book, however, lies in the individual chapters covering an expanded range of topics including arrhythmias, atrioventricular (AV) blocks, 12-lead ECGs, right-sided ECGs, posterior ECGs, acute coronary syndromes, Wellen's syndrome, pericarditis, electrolyte imbalances, bundle-branch blocks and fascicular blocks, atrial enlargement and ventricular hypertrophy, narrow versus wide complex tachycardias, permanent and temporary pacing, biventricular pacing, implantable cardioverter-defibrillators, radiofrequency catheter ablation, and ventricular assist devices. Each chapter comprehensively covers the cause of the disturbance, clinical significance of the disorder, expected ECG characteristics, and recommended treatment modalities. The last chapter includes practice rhythm strips, and the appendices cover clinically relevant features, such as:

- rapid reference to major arrhythmias
- cardiac drug overview.

Another major feature of *Interpreting Difficult ECGs* is the use of icons to highlight critical concepts. For instance, *Red flag* alerts the reader to key material; *Look-alikes* identify two rhythms that share similar features and can be tricky to distinguish from each other; *Life-threatening* indicates rhythms that require immediate treatment; and *Lead of choice* explains which lead system is best suited to monitoring a particular arrhythmia. For example, lead II is used to monitor a patient with a narrow QRS complex tachycardia. The book is enhanced by the use of color pages and more than 200 illustrations and tables.

In sum, *Interpreting Difficult ECGs: A Rapid Reference* is an excellent, advanced ECG interpretation book that will take the practicing nurse, advanced practice nurse, and students of all levels from the basics of arrhythmia recognition through 12-lead ECG interpretation and beyond. It combines clinically relevant assessment parameters, ECG interpretation, and current treatment modalities in a well-organized, evidence-based book that's a desirable addition to one's practice armamentaria.

Theresa Pluth Yeo, RN, MSN, MPH, ACNP
Assistant Professor
The Johns Hopkins University
School of Nursing
Baltimore

Part I
Reviewing fundamentals

1 Cardiac anatomy and physiology

Correct electrocardiogram (ECG) interpretation provides an important challenge to any practitioner. With a good understanding of ECGs, you'll be better able to provide expert care to your patients. For example, when you're caring for a patient with an arrhythmia or a myocardial infarction, an ECG waveform can help you quickly assess his condition and, if necessary, begin lifesaving interventions.

To build ECG skills, begin with the basics covered in this chapter — an overview of the heart's anatomy and physiology and electrical conduction system.

■ Cardiac anatomy

The heart is a hollow, muscular organ that works like a mechanical pump. It delivers oxygenated blood to the body through the arteries. When blood returns through the veins, the heart pumps it to the lungs to be reoxygenated.

LOCATION AND STRUCTURE

The heart lies obliquely in the chest, behind the sternum in the mediastinal cavity, or *mediastinum*. It's located between the lungs, in front of the spine. The top of the heart, called the *base,* lies just below the second rib. The bottom of the heart, called the *apex,* tilts forward and down toward the left side of the body and rests on the diaphragm. (See *Where the heart lies.*)

The heart varies in size, depending on the person's body size, but is roughly 5″ (12 cm) long and 3½″ (9 cm) wide, or about the size of the person's fist. The heart's weight, typically 9 to 12 oz (255 to 340 g), varies depending on the individual's size, age, gender, and athletic conditioning. An athlete's heart usually weighs more than average, whereas an elderly person's heart weighs less.

An infant's heart is positioned more horizontally in the chest cavity than an adult's. As a result, the apex is positioned at the fourth left inter-

Where the heart lies

The heart lies within the mediastinum, a cavity that contains the tissues and organs separating the two pleural sacs. In most people, two-thirds of the heart extends to the left of the body's midline.

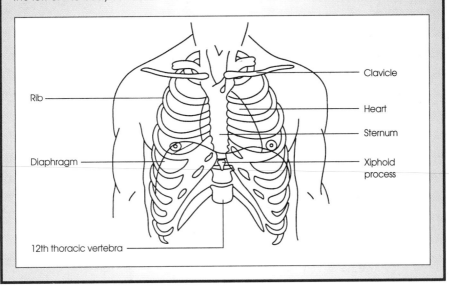

Clavicle

Rib

Heart

Sternum

Diaphragm

Xiphoid process

12th thoracic vertebra

costal space. Until age 4, a child's apical impulse is left of the midclavicular line. By age 7, his heart is located in the same position as an adult's heart is.

As a person ages, his heart usually becomes slightly smaller and loses its contractile strength and efficiency. In persons with hypertension, a moderate increase in left ventricular wall thickness may occur. As the myocardium of the aging heart becomes more irritable, extrasystoles may occur, along with sinus arrhythmias and sinus bradycardias. In addition, increased fibrous tissue infiltrates the sinoatrial (SA) node and internodal atrial tracts, which may cause atrial fibrillation and flutter.

By age 70, cardiac output at rest has diminished by 30% to 35% in many people.

HEART WALL

The heart wall, which encases the heart, is made up of three layers: epicardium, myocardium, and endocardium. The *epicardium*, the outermost layer, consists of squamous epithelial cells overlying connective tissue. The *myocardium*, the middle and thickest layer, makes up the largest portion of the heart's wall. This layer of muscle tissue contracts with each heartbeat. The endocardium, the heart wall's innermost layer, consists of a thin layer of endothelial tissue that lines the heart valves and chambers. (See *Layers of the heart wall*, page 4.)

Layers of the heart wall

This cross section of the heart wall shows its various layers.

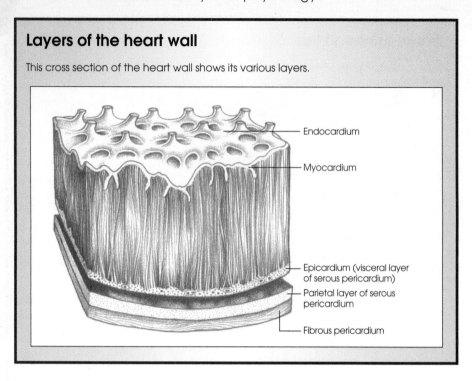

— Endocardium

— Myocardium

— Epicardium (visceral layer of serous pericardium)

— Parietal layer of serous pericardium

— Fibrous pericardium

The *pericardium* is a fluid-filled sac that envelops the heart and acts as a tough, protective covering. It consists of the fibrous pericardium and the serous pericardium. The fibrous pericardium is composed of tough, white, fibrous tissue, which fits loosely around the heart and protects it. The serous pericardium, the thin, smooth, inner portion, has two layers:

- parietal layer, which lines the inside of the fibrous pericardium
- visceral layer, which adheres to the surface of the heart.

The pericardial space separates the visceral and parietal layers and contains 10 to 30 ml of thin, clear, pericardial fluid, which lubricates the two surfaces and cushions the heart. Excess pericardial fluid, a condition called *pericardial effusion,* can compromise the heart's ability to pump blood.

HEART CHAMBERS

The heart contains four chambers — two atria and two ventricles. (See *Inside a normal heart.*) The right atrium lies in front of and to the right of the smaller but thicker-walled left atrium. An interatrial septum separates the two chambers and helps them contract. The right and left atria serve as volume reservoirs for blood being sent into the ventricles. The right atrium receives deoxygenated blood returning from the body through the inferior and superior venae cavae and from the heart through the coronary sinus. The left atrium receives oxygenated blood from the lungs through the four pulmonary veins. Contraction of the atria forces blood into the ventricles.

Inside a normal heart

This cross section shows the internal structure of a normal heart.

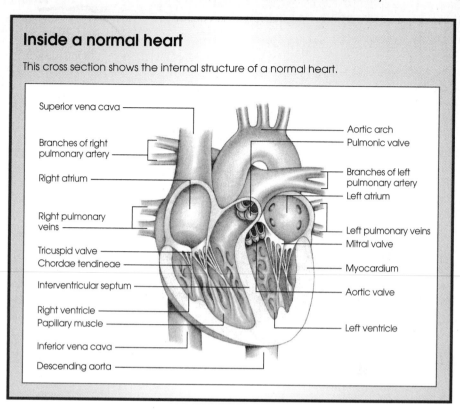

Superior vena cava

Branches of right pulmonary artery

Right atrium

Right pulmonary veins

Tricuspid valve

Chordae tendineae

Interventricular septum

Right ventricle

Papillary muscle

Inferior vena cava

Descending aorta

Aortic arch

Pulmonic valve

Branches of left pulmonary artery

Left atrium

Left pulmonary veins

Mitral valve

Myocardium

Aortic valve

Left ventricle

The right and left ventricles serve as the pumping chambers of the heart. The right ventricle lies behind the sternum and forms the largest part of the heart's sternocostal surface and inferior border. The right ventricle receives deoxygenated blood from the right atrium and pumps it through the pulmonary arteries to the lungs, where it's reoxygenated. The left ventricle forms the heart's apex, most of its left border, and most of its posterior and diaphragmatic surfaces. The left ventricle receives oxygenated blood from the left atrium and pumps it through the aorta into the systemic circulation. The interventricular septum separates the ventricles and helps them pump.

The thickness of a chamber's walls is determined by the amount of pressure needed to eject its blood. Because the atria act as reservoirs for the ventricles and pump the blood a shorter distance, their walls are considerably thinner than the walls of the ventricles. Likewise, the left ventricle has a much thicker wall than the right ventricle because the left ventricle pumps blood against the higher pressures in the aorta. The right ventricle pumps blood against the lower pressures in the pulmonary circulation.

HEART VALVES

The heart contains four valves — two atrioventricular (AV) valves (tricuspid and mitral) and two semilunar valves (aortic and pulmonic). Each valve consists of cusps, or *leaflets,* that open and close in response to pressure changes within the chambers they connect. The primary function of the valves is to keep blood flowing forward through the heart. When the valves close, they prevent backflow, or regurgitation, of blood from one chamber to another. Closure of the valves is associated with heart sounds.

The two AV valves are located between the atria and ventricles. The tricuspid valve, named for its three cusps, separates the right atrium from the right ventricle. The mitral valve, sometimes referred to as the *bicuspid valve* because of its two cusps, separates the left atrium from the left ventricle. Closure of the AV valves is associated with S_1, or the first heart sound.

The cusps of these valves are anchored to the papillary muscles of the ventricles by small tendinous cords called *chordae tendineae*. During ventricular contraction, the papillary muscles and chordae tendineae work together to prevent the cusps from bulging backward into the atria. Disruption of either structure may prevent complete valve closure, allowing blood to flow backward into the atria. This backward blood flow may cause a heart murmur.

The *semilunar valves* are so called because their three cusps resemble half moons. The pulmonic valve, located where the pulmonary artery meets the right ventricle, permits blood to flow from the right ventricle to the pulmonary artery and prevents backflow into the right ventricle. The aortic valve, located where the left ventricle meets the aorta, allows blood to flow from the left ventricle to the aorta and prevents blood backflow into the left ventricle.

Increased pressure within the ventricles during ventricular systole causes the pulmonic and aortic valves to open, allowing ejection of blood into the pulmonary and systemic circulation. Loss of pressure as the ventricular chambers empty causes the valves to close. Closure of the semilunar valves is associated with S_2, or the second heart sound.

BLOOD FLOW THROUGH THE HEART

Understanding the flow of blood through the heart is critical for understanding the overall functions of the heart and the way that changes in electrical activity affect peripheral blood flow. It's also important to remember that right- and left-sided heart events occur simultaneously.

Deoxygenated blood from the body returns to the heart through the inferior vena cava, superior vena cava, and coronary sinus and empties into the right atrium. The increasing volume of blood in the right atrium raises the pressure in that chamber above the pressure in the right ventricle. Then the tricuspid valve opens, allowing blood to flow into the right ventricle.

The right ventricle pumps blood through the pulmonic valve into the pulmonary arteries and lungs, where oxygen is picked up and excess carbon dioxide is released. From the lungs, the oxygenated blood flows through the pulmonary veins and into the left atrium. This completes a circuit called *pulmonic circulation*.

As the volume of blood in the left atrium increases, the pressure in the left atrium exceeds the pressure in the left ventricle. The mitral valve opens, allowing blood to flow into the left ventricle. The ventricle contracts and ejects the blood through the aortic valve into the aorta. The blood is distributed throughout the body, releasing oxygen to the cells and picking up carbon dioxide. Blood then returns to the right atrium through the veins, completing a circuit called *systemic circulation*.

CORONARY BLOOD SUPPLY

Like the brain and all other organs, the heart needs an adequate supply of oxygenated blood to survive. The main coronary arteries lie on the surface of the heart, with smaller arterial branches penetrating the surface into the cardiac muscle mass. The heart receives its blood supply almost entirely through these arteries. In fact, only a small percentage of the heart's endocardial surface can obtain sufficient amounts of nutrition directly from the blood in the cardiac chambers. (See *Vessels that supply the heart*, page 8.)

Understanding coronary blood flow can help you provide better care to a patient with coronary artery disease because you'll be able to predict which areas of the heart would be affected by a narrowing or occlusion of a particular coronary artery.

Coronary arteries

The left main and right coronary arteries arise from the coronary ostia, small orifices located just above the aortic valve cusps. The right coronary artery fills the groove between the atria and ventricles, giving rise to the acute marginal artery and ending as the posterior descending artery. The right coronary artery supplies blood to the right atrium, the right ventricle, and the inferior wall of the left ventricle. This artery also supplies blood to the SA node in about 50% of the population and to the AV node in 90% of the population. The posterior descending artery supplies the posterior wall of the left ventricle in 80% to 90% of the population.

The left main coronary artery varies in length from a few millimeters to a few centimeters. It splits into two major branches, the left anterior descending artery (also known as the *interventricular* artery) and the left circumflex artery. The left anterior descending artery runs down the anterior surface of the heart toward the apex. This artery and its branches — the diagonal arteries and the septal perforators — supply blood to the anterior wall of the left ventricle, the anterior interventricular septum, the bundle of His, the right bundle branch, and the anterior fasciculus of the left bundle branch.

The circumflex artery circles the left ventricle, ending on its posterior surface. The obtuse marginal artery arises from the circumflex artery. The circumflex artery provides oxygenated blood to the lateral wall of the left ventricle, the left atrium, the posterior wall of the left ventricle in

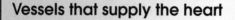

Vessels that supply the heart

The coronary circulation involves the arterial system of blood vessels, which supplies oxygenated blood to the heart, and the venous system, which removes oxygen-depleted blood from the heart.

ANTERIOR VIEW

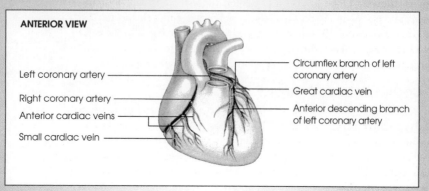

Left coronary artery

Right coronary artery

Anterior cardiac veins

Small cardiac vein

Circumflex branch of left coronary artery

Great cardiac vein

Anterior descending branch of left coronary artery

POSTERIOR VIEW

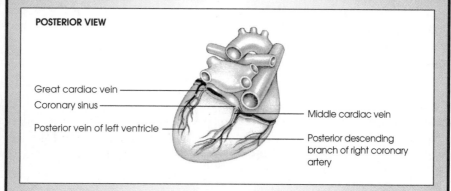

Great cardiac vein

Coronary sinus

Posterior vein of left ventricle

Middle cardiac vein

Posterior descending branch of right coronary artery

10% of the population, and the posterior fasciculus of the left bundle branch. In about 50% of the population, it supplies the SA node; in about 10% of the population, the AV node.

In most of the population, the right coronary artery is the dominant vessel, meaning that the right coronary artery supplies the posterior wall via the posterior descending artery. This system is described as *right coronary dominance* or a *dominant right coronary artery*. Likewise, patients in whom the left coronary artery supplies the posterior wall via the posterior descending artery, the terms *left coronary dominance* or a *dominant left coronary artery* are used.

When two or more arteries supply the same region, they usually connect through anastomoses, junctions that provide alternative routes of blood flow. This network of smaller arteries, called *collateral circulation*, provides blood to capillaries that directly feed the heart muscle. Collateral circulation becomes so strong in many patients that even if major coronary arteries become narrowed with plaque, collateral circulation can continue to supply blood to the heart.

Coronary artery blood flow

In contrast to the other vascular beds in the body, the heart receives its blood supply primarily during ventricular relaxation, or diastole, when the left ventricle is filling with blood. This effect results because the coronary ostia lie near the aortic valve and become partially occluded when the aortic valve opens during ventricular contraction or systole. However, when the aortic valve closes, the ostia are unobstructed, allowing blood to fill the coronary arteries. Because diastole is the time when the coronary arteries receive their blood supply, anything that shortens diastole, such as periods of increased heart rate or tachycardia, also decreases coronary blood flow.

In addition, the left ventricular muscle compresses the intramuscular vessels during systole. During diastole, the cardiac muscle relaxes, and blood flow through the left ventricular capillaries is no longer obstructed.

Cardiac veins

Similar to other parts of the body, the heart has its own veins, which remove oxygen-depleted blood from the myocardium. About 75% of the total coronary venous blood flow leaves the left ventricle by way of the coronary sinus, an enlarged vessel that returns blood to the right atrium. Most of the venous blood from the right ventricle flows directly into the right atrium through the small anterior cardiac veins, not by way of the coronary sinus. A small amount of coronary blood flows back into the heart through the thebesian veins, minute veins that empty directly into all chambers of the heart.

■ Cardiac physiology

In this section, you'll find descriptions of the cardiac cycle; cardiac muscle innervation; depolarization and repolarization; and normal and abnormal impulse conduction.

THE CARDIAC CYCLE

The cardiac cycle includes the cardiac events that occur from the beginning of one heartbeat to the beginning of the next. The cardiac cycle consists of ventricular diastole, or relaxation, and ventricular systole, or contraction. During ventricular diastole, blood flows from the atria through the open tricuspid and mitral valves into the relaxed ventricles. The aortic and pulmonic valves are closed during ventricular diastole. (See *Phases of the cardiac cycle*, page 10.)

Phases of the cardiac cycle

The cardiac cycle consists of these phases:

1. Isovolumetric ventricular contraction — In response to ventricular depolarization, tension in the ventricles increases. The rise in pressure within the ventricles leads to closure of the mitral and tricuspid valves. The pulmonic and aortic valves stay closed during the entire phase.

2. Ventricular ejection — When ventricular pressure exceeds aortic and pulmonary artery pressures, the aortic and pulmonic valves open and the ventricles eject blood.

3. Isovolumetric relaxation — When ventricular pressure falls below the pressures in the aorta and pulmonary artery, the aortic and pulmonic valves close. All valves are closed during this phase. Atrial diastole occurs as blood fills the atria.

4. Ventricular filling — Atrial pressure exceeds ventricular pressure, which causes the mitral and tricuspid valves to open. Blood then flows passively into the ventricles. About 70% of ventricular filling takes place during this phase.

5. Atrial systole — Known as the *atrial kick,* atrial systole (coinciding with late ventricular diastole) supplies the ventricles with the remaining 30% of the blood for each heartbeat.

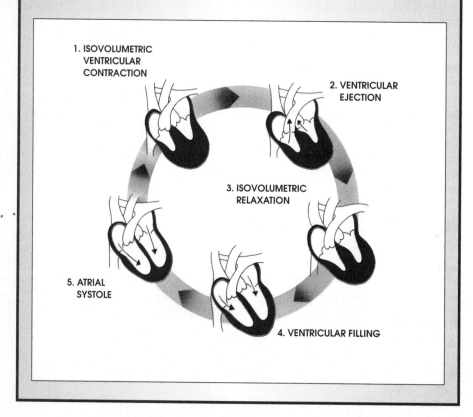

1. ISOVOLUMETRIC VENTRICULAR CONTRACTION

2. VENTRICULAR EJECTION

3. ISOVOLUMETRIC RELAXATION

5. ATRIAL SYSTOLE

4. VENTRICULAR FILLING

During diastole, about 75% of the blood flows passively from the atria through the open tricuspid and mitral valves and into the ventricles even before the atria contract. Atrial contraction, or *atrial kick* as it's some-

Preload and afterload

Preload refers to a passive stretching that blood exerts on the ventricular muscle fibers at the end of diastole. According to Starling's law, the more the cardiac muscles are stretched in diastole, the more forcefully they contract in systole.

Afterload refers to the pressure that the ventricles need to generate to overcome higher pressure in the aorta to eject blood into the systemic circulation. This systemic vascular resistance corresponds to the systemic systolic pressure.

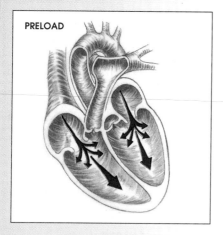

PRELOAD

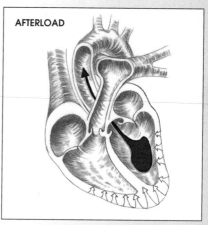

AFTERLOAD

times called, contributes another 25% to ventricular filling. Loss of effective atrial contraction occurs with some arrhythmias, such as atrial fibrillation. This loss results in a reduction in cardiac output.

During ventricular systole, the mitral and tricuspid valves are closed as the relaxed atria fill with blood. As ventricular pressure rises, the aortic and pulmonic valves open. The ventricles contract, and blood is ejected into the pulmonic and systemic circulation.

CARDIAC OUTPUT

Cardiac output is the amount of blood the left ventricle pumps into the aorta per minute. Cardiac output is measured by multiplying heart rate times stroke volume. Stroke volume refers to the amount of blood ejected with each ventricular contraction and is usually about 70 ml.

Normal cardiac output is 4 to 8 L/minute, depending on body size. The heart pumps only as much blood as the body requires, based on metabolic requirements. During exercise, for example, the heart increases cardiac output accordingly.

Three factors determine stroke volume: preload, afterload, and myocardial contractility. (See *Preload and afterload.*) Preload is the degree of stretch, or tension, on the muscle fibers when they begin to contract. It's usually considered to be the end-diastolic pressure when the ventricle has filled.

Afterload is the load (or amount of pressure) the left ventricle must work against to eject blood during systole and corresponds to the systolic pressure. The greater this resistance is, the greater the heart's workload. Afterload is also called the *systemic vascular resistance*.

Myocardial contractility is the ventricle's ability to contract, which is determined by the degree of muscle fiber stretch at the end of diastole. The more the muscle fibers stretch during ventricular filling, up to an optimal length, the more forceful the contraction.

AUTONOMIC INNERVATION OF THE HEART

The two branches of the autonomic nervous system — the sympathetic (or adrenergic) nervous system and the parasympathetic (or cholinergic) nervous system — abundantly supply the heart. Sympathetic fibers innervate all the areas of the heart, whereas parasympathetic fibers primarily innervate the SA and AV nodes.

Sympathetic nerve stimulation causes the release of norepinephrine, which increases the heart rate by increasing SA node discharge, accelerates AV node conduction time, and increases the force of myocardial contraction and cardiac output.

Parasympathetic (vagal) stimulation causes the release of acetylcholine, which produces the opposite effects. The rate of SA node discharge is decreased, thus slowing heart rate and conduction through the AV node, and reducing cardiac output.

TRANSMISSION OF ELECTRICAL IMPULSES

For the heart to contract and pump blood to the rest of the body, an electrical stimulus needs to occur first. Generation and transmission of electrical impulses depend on the four key characteristics of cardiac cells: automaticity, excitability, conductivity, and contractility.

Automaticity refers to a cell's ability to spontaneously initiate an electrical impulse. Pacemaker cells usually possess this ability. *Excitability* results from ion shifts across the cell membrane and refers to the cell's ability to respond to an electrical stimulus. *Conductivity* is the ability of a cell to transmit an electrical impulse from one cell to another. *Contractility* refers to the cell's ability to contract after receiving a stimulus by shortening and lengthening its muscle fibers.

It's important to remember that the first three characteristics are electrical properties of the cells, whereas contractility represents a mechanical response to the electrical activity. Of the four characteristics, automaticity has the greatest effect on the genesis of cardiac rhythms.

DEPOLARIZATION AND REPOLARIZATION

As impulses are transmitted, cardiac cells undergo cycles of depolarization and repolarization. (See *Depolarization-repolarization cycle.*) Cardiac cells at rest are considered polarized, meaning that no electrical activity takes place. Cell membranes separate different concentrations of ions, such as sodium and potassium, and create a more negative charge inside

Depolarization-repolarization cycle

The depolarization-repolarization cycle consists of these phases.

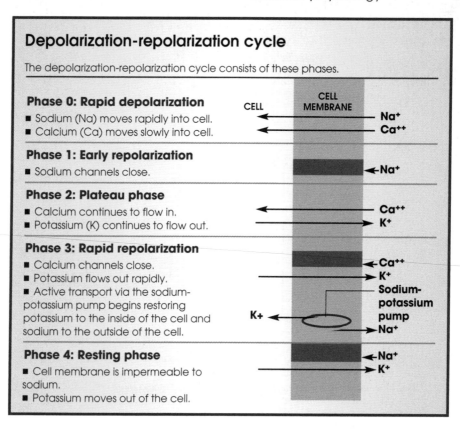

Phase 0: Rapid depolarization
- Sodium (Na) moves rapidly into cell.
- Calcium (Ca) moves slowly into cell.

Phase 1: Early repolarization
- Sodium channels close.

Phase 2: Plateau phase
- Calcium continues to flow in.
- Potassium (K) continues to flow out.

Phase 3: Rapid repolarization
- Calcium channels close.
- Potassium flows out rapidly.
- Active transport via the sodium-potassium pump begins restoring potassium to the inside of the cell and sodium to the outside of the cell.

Phase 4: Resting phase
- Cell membrane is impermeable to sodium.
- Potassium moves out of the cell.

the cell. This phenomenon is called the *resting potential.* After a stimulus occurs, ions cross the cell membrane and cause an action potential, or cell depolarization. When a cell is fully depolarized, it attempts to return to its resting state in a process called *repolarization.* Electrical charges in the cell reverse and return to normal.

A cycle of depolarization-repolarization consists of five phases — 0 through 4. The action potential is represented by a curve that shows voltage changes during the five phases. (See *Action potential curves,* page 14.)

During phase 0 (or rapid depolarization), the cell receives a stimulus, usually from a neighboring cell. The cell becomes more permeable to sodium, the inside of the cell becomes less negative, the cell is depolarized, and myocardial contraction occurs. In phase 1 (or early repolarization), sodium stops flowing into the cell, and the transmembrane potential falls slightly. Phase 2 (the plateau phase) is a prolonged period of slow repolarization, when little change occurs in the cell's transmembrane potential.

During phases 1 and 2 and at the beginning of phase 3, the cardiac cell is said to be in its absolute refractory period. During that period, no stimulus — no matter how strong — can excite the cell.

Action potential curves

An action potential curve shows the changes in a cell's electrical charge during the five phases of the depolarization-repolarization cycle. These graphs show electrical changes for nonpacemaker and pacemaker cells.

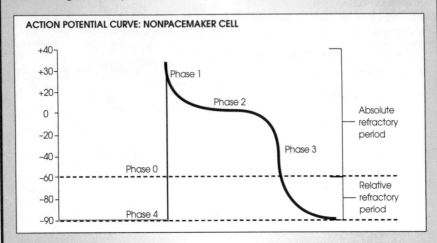

ACTION POTENTIAL CURVE: NONPACEMAKER CELL

As the graph below shows, the action potential curve for pacemaker cells, such as those in the sinoatrial node, differs from that of other myocardial cells. Pacemaker cells have a resting membrane potential of –60 mV (instead of –90 mV), and they begin to depolarize spontaneously. Called *diastolic depolarization,* this effect results primarily from calcium and sodium leakage into the cell.

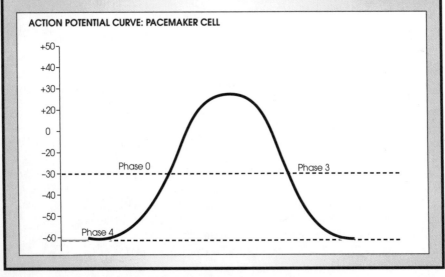

ACTION POTENTIAL CURVE: PACEMAKER CELL

Phase 3 (or rapid repolarization) occurs as the cell returns to its original state. During the last half of this phase, when the cell is in its relative refractory period, a strong stimulus can depolarize it.

Phase 4 is the resting phase of the action potential. By the end of phase 4, the cell is ready for another stimulus.

The electrical activity of the heart is represented on an ECG. Keep in mind that the ECG represents only electrical activity, not the mechanical activity or actual pumping of the heart.

ELECTRICAL CONDUCTION SYSTEM OF THE HEART

After depolarization and repolarization occur, the resulting electrical impulse travels through the heart along a pathway called the *conduction system*. (See *Cardiac conduction system*, page 16.)

Impulses travel out from the SA node and through the internodal tracts, and the interatrial tract (Bachmann's bundle) and to the AV node. From there, they travel through the bundle of His, the bundle branches, and finally to the Purkinje fibers.

The SA node, located in the right atrium where the superior vena cava joins the atrial tissue mass, is the heart's main pacemaker. Under resting conditions, the SA node generates impulses 60 to 100 beats/minute. When initiated, the impulses follow a specific path through the heart. Electrical impulses normally don't travel in a backward or retrograde direction because when the cells are activated they can't respond to another stimulus immediately after depolarization.

From the SA node, an impulse travels through the right and left atria. In the right atrium, the impulse is likely transmitted along three internodal tracts. These tracts include the anterior, the middle (or Wenckebach's), and the posterior (or Thorel's) internodal tracts. The impulse travels through the left atrium via Bachmann's bundle, the interatrial tract of tissue extending from the SA node to the left atrium. Impulse transmission through the right and left atria occurs so rapidly that the atria contract almost simultaneously.

Conduction to the ventricles

The AV node is located in the inferior right atrium, near the ostium of the coronary sinus. Although the AV node has no pacemaker cells, the tissue surrounding it, referred to as *junctional tissue,* contains pacemaker cells that can fire at a rate of 40 to 60 beats/minute. As the AV node conducts the atrial impulse to the ventricles, it causes a 0.04-second delay. This delay allows the ventricles to complete their filling phase as the atria contract. It also allows the cardiac muscle to stretch to its fullest for peak cardiac output.

Rapid conduction then resumes through the bundle of His, which divides into the right and left bundle branches and extends down either side of the interventricular septum. The right bundle branch extends down the right side of the interventricular septum and through the right ventricle. The left bundle branch extends down the left side of the interventricular septum and through the left ventricle. As a pacemaker site, the bundle of His has a firing rate between 40 and 60 beats/minute. The bundle of His usually fires when the SA node fails to generate an im-

Cardiac conduction system

The conduction system of the heart, as shown below, begins with the heart's dominant pacemaker, the sinoatrial (SA) node. The intrinsic rate of the SA node is 60 to 100 beats/minute. When an impulse leaves the SA node, it travels through the atria along Bachmann's bundle and the internodal pathways, on its way to the atrioventricular (AV) node and ventricles.

   After the impulse passes through the AV node, it travels to the ventricles, first down the bundle of His, then along the bundle branches, and finally down the Purkinje fibers. Pacemaker cells in the junctional tissue and Purkinje fibers of the ventricles normally remain dormant because they receive impulses from the SA node. They initiate an impulse only when they don't receive one from the SA node. The intrinsic rate of the AV junction is 40 to 60 beats/minute; the intrinsic rate of the ventricles, 20 to 40 beats/minute.

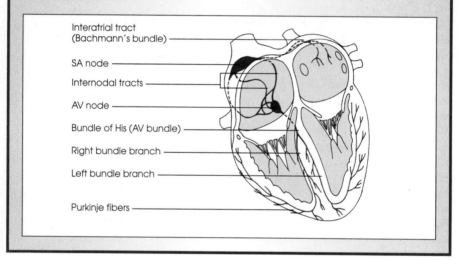

Interatrial tract
(Bachmann's bundle)

SA node

Internodal tracts

AV node

Bundle of His (AV bundle)

Right bundle branch

Left bundle branch

Purkinje fibers

pulse at a normal rate or when the impulse fails to reach the AV junction.

   The left bundle branch then splits into two branches, or *fasciculations*. The left anterior fasciculus extends through the anterior portion of the left ventricle. The left posterior fasciculus extends through the lateral and posterior portions of the left ventricle. Impulses travel much faster down the left bundle branch, which feeds the larger, thicker-walled left ventricle, than they do down the right bundle branch, which feeds the smaller, thinner-walled right ventricle. The difference in the conduction speed allows both ventricles to contract simultaneously. The entire network of specialized nervous tissue that extends through the ventricles is known as the *His-Purkinje system*.

   Purkinje fibers comprise a diffuse muscle fiber network beneath the endocardium that transmits impulses quicker than any other part of the conduction system does. This pacemaker site usually doesn't fire unless the SA and AV nodes fail to generate an impulse or the normal impulse is blocked in both bundle branches. The automatic firing rate of the Purkinje fibers ranges from 20 to 40 beats/minute. In children younger than age 3, the AV junction may discharge impulses at a rate of 50 to 80 times per minute; the Purkinje fibers may discharge at a rate of 40 to 50 times per minute.

ABNORMAL IMPULSE CONDUCTION

Causes of abnormal impulse conduction include altered automaticity, retrograde conduction of impulses, reentry abnormalities, and ectopy.

Automaticity, a special characteristic of pacemaker cells, allows them to generate electrical impulses spontaneously. If a cell's automaticity is increased or decreased, an arrhythmia — or abnormality in the cardiac rhythm — can occur. Tachycardia and premature beats are commonly caused by an increase in the automaticity of pacemaker cells below the SA node. Likewise, a decrease in automaticity of cells in the SA node can cause the development of bradycardia or escape rhythms generated by lower pacemaker sites.

When the electrical impulse is initiated at or below the AV node, it may be transmitted backward toward the atria. This backward, or retrograde, conduction usually takes longer than normal conduction and can cause the atria and ventricles to lose synchrony.

Reentry occurs when cardiac tissue is activated two or more times by the same impulse, for example, when conduction speed is slowed or when the refractory periods for neighboring cells occur at different times. Impulses are delayed long enough that cells have time to repolarize. In those cases, the active impulse reenters the same area and produces another impulse.

Injured pacemaker or nonpacemaker cells may partially depolarize, rather than fully depolarizing. Partial depolarization can lead to spontaneous or secondary depolarization, repetitive ectopic firings called *triggered activity*.

The resultant depolarization is called *afterdepolarization*. Early afterdepolarization occurs before the cell is fully repolarized and can be caused by hypokalemia, slow pacing rates, or drug toxicity. If it occurs after the cell has been fully repolarized, it's called *delayed afterdepolarization*. These problems can be caused by digoxin toxicity, hypercalcemia, or increased catecholamine release. Atrial or ventricular tachycardias may result.

Part II
Interpreting rhythm strips

2 *Reading ECGs*

One of the most valuable diagnostic tools available, an electrocardiogram (ECG) records the heart's electrical activity as waveforms. By interpreting these waveforms accurately, you can identify rhythm disturbances, conduction abnormalities, and electrolyte imbalances. An ECG aids in diagnosing and monitoring conditions, such as acute coronary syndromes and pericarditis.

To interpret an ECG correctly, you must first recognize its key components. Next, you need to analyze them separately. Then you can put your findings together to reach a conclusion about the heart's electrical activity. This chapter explains that analytic process, beginning with some fundamental information about electrocardiography.

The heart's electrical activity produces currents that radiate through the surrounding tissue to the skin. When electrodes are attached to the skin, they sense those electrical currents and transmit them to the electrocardiograph. This electrical activity is transformed into waveforms that represent the heart's depolarization-repolarization cycle.

Myocardial depolarization occurs when a wave of stimulation passes through the heart and causes the heart muscle to contract. Repolarization is the relaxation phase. An ECG shows the precise sequence of electrical events occurring in the cardiac cells throughout that process and identifies rhythm disturbances and conduction abnormalities.

■ *Leads and planes*

Because the electrical currents from the heart radiate to the skin in many directions, electrodes are placed at different locations to obtain a total picture of the heart's electrical activity. The ECG can then record information from different perspectives, which are called *leads* and *planes*.

LEADS
A lead provides a view of the heart's electrical activity between two points, or poles. Each lead consists of one positive and one negative pole.

Current direction and waveform deflection

This illustration shows possible directions of electrical current and the corresponding waveform deflections. The direction of the electrical current through the heart determines the upward or downward deflection of an electrocardiogram waveform.

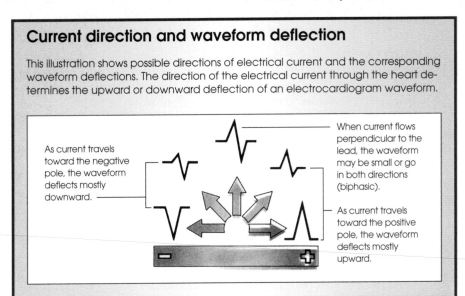

As current travels toward the negative pole, the waveform deflects mostly downward.

When current flows perpendicular to the lead, the waveform may be small or go in both directions (biphasic).

As current travels toward the positive pole, the waveform deflects mostly upward.

Between the two poles lies an imaginary line representing the lead's axis, a term that refers to the direction of the current moving through the heart. Because each lead measures the heart's electrical potential from different directions, each generates its own characteristic tracing. (See *Current direction and waveform deflection.*)

The direction in which the electric current flows determines how the waveforms appear on the ECG tracing. When the current flows along the axis toward the positive pole of the electrode, the waveform deflects upward and is called a *positive deflection*. When the current flows away from the positive pole, the waveform deflects downward, below the baseline, and is called a *negative deflection*. When the current flows perpendicular to the axis, the wave may go in both directions or may be unusually small. When electrical activity is absent or too small to measure, the waveform is a straight line, also called an *isoelectric deflection*.

PLANES

A plane is a cross section of the heart, which provides a different view of the heart's electrical activity. In the frontal plane — a vertical cut through the middle of the heart from top to bottom — electrical activity is viewed from right and left. The six limb leads are viewed from the frontal plane.

In the horizontal plane — a transverse cut through the middle of the heart dividing it into upper and lower portions — electrical activity can be viewed moving anteriorly and posteriorly. The six precordial leads are viewed from the horizontal plane.

■ Types of ECG recordings

The two main types of ECG recordings are the 12-lead ECG and the single-lead ECG, commonly known as a *rhythm strip*. Both types give valuable information about the heart's electrical activity.

12-LEAD ECG

A 12-lead ECG records information from 12 different views of the heart and provides a complete picture of electrical activity. These 12 views are obtained by placing electrodes on the patient's limbs and chest. The limb leads and the chest, or *precordial*, leads reflect information from the different planes of the heart.

Different leads provide different information. The six limb leads — I, II, III, augmented vector right (aV_R), augmented vector left (aV_L), and augmented vector foot (aV_F) — provide information about the heart's frontal plane. Leads I, II, and III require a negative and positive electrode for monitoring, which makes these leads bipolar. The augmented leads — aV_R, aV_L, and aV_F — are unipolar, meaning they need only a positive electrode.

The six precordial, or V, leads — V_1, V_2, V_3, V_4, V_5, and V_6 — provide information about the heart's horizontal plane. Like the augmented leads, the precordial leads are unipolar, requiring only a positive electrode. The negative pole of these leads, which is in the center of the heart, is calculated with the ECG.

SINGLE-LEAD ECG

Single-lead monitoring provides continuous information about the heart's electrical activity and is used to monitor cardiac status. Chest electrodes pick up the heart's electrical activity for display on the monitor. The monitor also displays heart rate and other measurements and prints out strips of cardiac rhythms.

Commonly monitored leads include the bipolar leads I, II, and III. Two other leads, MCL_1 and MCL_6, may also be used. MCL stands for *modified chest lead*. These leads are similar to the unipolar leads V_1 and V_6 of the 12-lead ECG; MCL_1 and MCL_6, however, are bipolar leads.

■ ECG monitoring systems

The type of ECG monitoring system used — hardwire monitoring or telemetry — depends on the patient's clinical status. With hardwire monitoring, the electrodes are connected directly to the cardiac monitor. Most hardwire monitors are mounted permanently on a shelf or wall near the patient's bed. Some monitors are mounted on an I.V. pole for portability, and some include a defibrillator.

The monitor provides a continuous cardiac rhythm display and transmits the ECG tracing to a console at the nurses' station. Both the moni-

tor and the console have alarms and can print rhythm strips to show ectopic beats, for example, or other arrhythmias. Hardwire monitors also
have the ability to track pulse oximetry, blood pressure, hemodynamic
measurements, and other parameters through various attachments to
the patient.

Hardwire monitoring is generally used in critical care units and emergency departments because it permits continuous observation of one or
more patients from more than one area in the unit. However, this type of
monitoring does have disadvantages, including limited mobility because
the patient is tethered to a monitor.

With telemetry monitoring, the patient carries a small, battery-
powered transmitter that sends electrical signals to another location,
where the signals are displayed on a monitor screen. This type of ECG
monitoring frees the patient from cumbersome wires and cables and
protects him from the electrical leakage and accidental shock occasionally associated with hardwire monitoring.

Telemetry monitoring still requires skin electrodes to be placed on the
patient's chest. Each electrode is connected by a thin wire to a small
transmitter box carried in a pocket or pouch. Telemetry monitoring is especially useful for detecting arrhythmias that occur at rest or during
sleep, exercise, or stressful situations. Most systems, however, can monitor only heart rate and rhythm.

■ *Electrode placement*

Electrode placement is different for each lead, and different leads provide different views of the heart. A lead may be chosen to highlight a particular part of the ECG complex or the electrical events of a specific area
of the heart.

Although leads II, V_1, and V_6 are among the most commonly used
leads for continuous monitoring, lead placement is varied according to
the patient's clinical status. If your monitoring system has the capability,
you may also monitor the patient in more than one lead. (See *Dual-lead
monitoring,* page 24.)

STANDARD LIMB LEADS

All standard limb leads or bipolar limb leads have a third electrode,
known as the *ground,* which is placed on the chest to prevent electrical
interference from appearing on the ECG recording.

Lead I provides a view of the heart that shows current moving from
right to left. Because current flows from negative to positive, the positive
electrode for this lead is placed on the left arm or on the left side of the
chest; the negative electrode is placed on the right arm. Lead I produces
a positive deflection on ECG tracings and is helpful in monitoring atrial
rhythms.

Lead II produces a positive deflection. The positive electrode is placed
on the patient's left leg and the negative electrode on the right arm. For

Dual-lead monitoring

Monitoring in two leads provides a more complete picture than monitoring in one does. Therefore, if it's available, dual-lead monitoring should be used to detect ectopy or aberrant rhythms.

With simultaneous dual monitoring, the first lead — typically designated as the primary lead (lead II) — is usually reviewed for arrhythmias. The second lead (lead V_1) helps detect ectopic beats or aberrant rhythms. Leads II and V_1 are the leads most commonly monitored simultaneously.

LEAD II

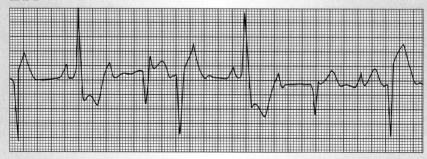

LEAD V_1

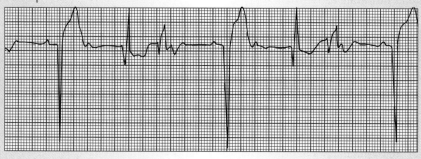

continuous monitoring, place the electrodes on the patient's torso for convenience, with the positive electrode below the lowest palpable rib at the left midclavicular line and the negative electrode below the right clavicle. The current travels down and to the left in this lead. Lead II tends to produce a positive, high-voltage deflection, resulting in tall P, R, and T waves. This lead is commonly used for routine monitoring and is useful for detecting sinus node and atrial arrhythmias and for monitoring the inferior wall of the left ventricle.

Lead III usually produces a positive deflection. The positive electrode is placed on the left leg and the negative electrode on the left arm. Along with lead II, this lead is useful for detecting changes associated with an inferior wall of the left ventricle.

The axes of the three bipolar limb leads — I, II, and III — form a triangle around the heart and provide a frontal plane view of the heart. (See *Einthoven's triangle.*)

Einthoven's triangle

The axes of the three bipolar limb leads (I, II, and III) form a triangle, known as *Einthoven's triangle*. Because the electrodes for these leads are about equidistant from the heart, the triangle is equilateral.

The axis of lead I extends from shoulder to shoulder, with the right arm lead being the negative electrode and the left arm lead being the positive electrode. The axis of lead II runs from the negative right arm lead electrode to the positive left leg lead electrode. The axis of lead III extends from the negative left arm lead electrode to the positive left leg lead electrode.

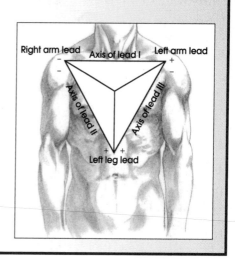

AUGMENTED UNIPOLAR LEADS

Leads aV_R, aV_L, and aV_F are called *augmented leads* because the ECG enhances the small waveforms that would normally appear from these unipolar leads.

In lead aV_R, the positive electrode is placed on the right arm and produces a negative deflection because the heart's electrical activity moves away from the lead. In lead aV_L, the positive electrode is on the left arm and usually produces a positive deflection on the ECG. In lead aV_F, the positive electrode is on the left leg (despite the name aV_F) and produces a positive deflection. These three limb leads also provide a view of the heart's frontal plane.

PRECORDIAL UNIPOLAR LEADS

The six unipolar *precordial leads* are placed in sequence across the chest and provide a view of the heart's horizontal plane. (See *Precordial views*, page 26.)

The precordial lead V_1 electrode is placed on the right side of the sternum at the fourth intercostal rib space.

Lead V_2 is placed to the left of the sternum at the fourth intercostal space.

Lead V_3 goes between V_2 and V_4 at the fifth intercostal space. Leads V_1, V_2, and V_3 are biphasic, with positive and negative deflections.

Lead V_4 is placed at the fifth intercostal space at the midclavicular line and produces a positive deflection.

Lead V_5 is placed between leads V_4 and V_6 anterior to the axillary line. Lead V_5 produces a positive deflection on the ECG.

Lead V_6, the last of the precordial leads, is placed level with lead V_4 at the midaxillary line. Lead V_6 produces a positive deflection on the ECG.

Precordial views

These illustrations show the different views of the heart obtained from each precordial (chest) lead.

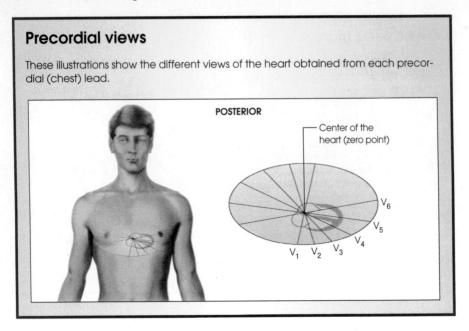

These precordial leads are useful in monitoring ventricular arrhythmias, ST-segment changes, and bundle-branch blocks.

MODIFIED CHEST LEADS

The modification of the chest lead occurs because a negative electrode is placed on the left side of the chest, rather than having the center of the heart function as the negative lead. MCL_1 is created by placing the negative electrode on the left upper chest, the positive electrode on the right side of the heart, and the ground electrode usually on the right upper chest. The MCL_1 lead most closely approximates the ECG pattern produced by the chest lead V_1.

When the positive electrode is on the right side of the heart and the electrical current travels toward the left ventricle, the waveform has a negative deflection. As a result, ectopic, or abnormal, beats deflect in a positive direction.

Choose MCL_1 to assess QRS-complex arrhythmias as a bipolar substitute for V_1. You can use this lead to monitor premature ventricular beats and to distinguish different types of tachycardia, such as ventricular and supraventricular tachycardia. MCL_1 can also be used to assess bundle-branch defects and P-wave changes and to confirm pacemaker wire placement.

MCL_6 is an alternative to MCL_1 and most closely approximates the ECG pattern produced by the chest lead V_6. Like MCL_1, it monitors ventricular conduction changes. The positive lead in MCL_6 is placed at the midaxillary line of the left fifth intercostal space, the negative electrode below the left shoulder, and the ground below the right shoulder.

ECG grid

This electrocardiogram (ECG) grid shows the horizontal axis and vertical axis and their respective measurement values.

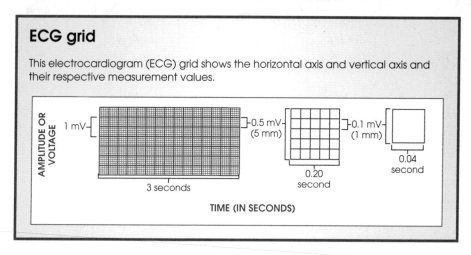

■ *Examining the ECG grid*

Waveforms produced by the heart's electrical current are recorded on graphed ECG paper by a heated stylus. ECG paper consists of horizontal and vertical lines forming a grid. A piece of ECG paper is called an *ECG strip* or *tracing*. (See *ECG grid.*)

The horizontal axis of the ECG strip represents time. Each small block equals 0.04 second, and five small blocks form a large block, which equals 0.2 second. This time increment is determined by multiplying 0.04 second (for one small block) by five, the number of small blocks that make up a large block. Five large blocks equal 1 second (5 × 0.2). When measuring or calculating a patient's heart rate, a 6-second strip consisting of 30 large blocks is usually used.

The ECG strip's vertical axis measures amplitude in millimeters (mm) or electrical voltage in millivolts (mV). Each small block represents 1 mm or 0.1 mV; each large block, 5 mm or 0.5 mV. To determine the amplitude of a wave, segment, or interval, count the number of small blocks from the baseline to the highest or lowest point of the wave, segment, or interval.

■ *ECG waveform components*

An ECG complex represents the heart's electrical activity (depolarization-repolarization cycle) occurring in one cardiac cycle. The ECG tracing consists of three basic waveforms: the P wave, the QRS complex, and the T wave. These units of electrical activity can be further broken down into these segments and intervals: the PR interval, the ST segment, and the QT interval.

In addition, a U wave may sometimes be present. The J point marks the end of the QRS complex and the beginning of the ST segment. (See *ECG waveform components.*)

The upward and downward movement of the ECG machine's stylus, which forms the various waves, reflects the directional flow of the heart's electrical impulse. When the electrodes are placed correctly, an upward deflection is positive and a downward deflection is negative. Between each cardiac cycle, when the heart's electrical activity is absent, the stylus on the ECG recorder returns to the baseline or isoelectric line and records a straight line.

P WAVE

The P wave is the first component of a normal ECG waveform. It represents atrial depolarization or conduction of an electrical impulse through the atria. When evaluating a P wave, look closely at its characteristics, especially its location, configuration, and deflection. A normal P wave has the following characteristics.

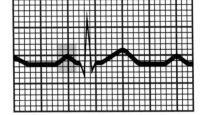

- Location: precedes the QRS complex
- Amplitude: 2 to 3 mm high
- Duration: 0.06 to 0.12 second
- Configuration: usually rounded and upright
- Deflection: positive or upright in leads I, II, aV_F, and V_2 to V_6; usually positive but may vary in leads III and aV_L; negative or inverted in lead aV_R; biphasic or variable in lead V_1

If the deflection and configuration of a P wave are normal — for example, if the P wave is upright in lead II and is rounded and smooth — and if the P wave precedes each QRS complex, you can assume that this electrical impulse originated in the sinoatrial (SA) node. The atria start to contract partway through the P wave, but you won't see this on the ECG. Remember, the ECG records only electrical activity, not mechanical activity or contraction.

Peaked, notched, or enlarged P waves may represent atrial hypertrophy or enlargement associated with chronic obstructive pulmonary disease, pulmonary emboli, valvular disease, or heart failure. Inverted P waves may signify retrograde or reverse conduction from the atrioventricular (AV) junction toward the atria. Whenever an upright sinus P wave becomes inverted, consider retrograde conduction and reverse conduction as possible conditions.

Varying P waves indicate that the impulse may be coming from different sites, as with a wandering pacemaker rhythm, irritable atrial tissue, or damage near the SA node. Absent P waves may signify impulse initiation by tissue other than the SA node, as with a junctional or atrial fibrillation rhythm. When a P wave doesn't precede the QRS complex, heart block may be present.

ECG waveform components

This illustration shows the components of a normal electrocardiogram (ECG) waveform.

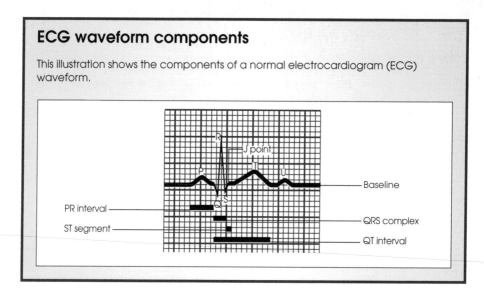

PR INTERVAL

The PR interval tracks the atrial impulse from the atria through the AV node, bundle of His, and right and left bundle branches. When evaluating a PR interval, look particularly at its duration. Changes in the PR interval indicate an altered impulse formation or a conduction delay, as seen in AV block. A normal PR interval has the following characteristics (amplitude, configuration, and deflection aren't measured).

■ Location: from the beginning of the P wave to the beginning of the QRS complex
■ Duration: 0.12 to 0.20 second

Short PR intervals (less than 0.12 second) indicate that the impulse originated somewhere other than the SA node. This variation is associated with junctional arrhythmias and preexcitation syndromes.

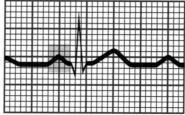

Prolonged PR intervals (greater than 0.20 second) may represent a conduction delay through the atria or AV junction resulting from digoxin toxicity or heart block — slowing related to ischemia or conduction tissue disease.

QRS COMPLEX

The QRS complex follows the P wave and represents depolarization of the ventricles, or *impulse conduction*. Immediately after the ventricles depolarize, as represented by the QRS complex, they contract. That contraction ejects blood from the ventricles and pumps it through the arteries, creating a pulse.

QRS waveform variety

These illustrations show the various configurations of QRS complexes. When documenting the QRS complex, use uppercase letters to indicate a wave with a normal or high amplitude (greater than 5 mm) and lowercase letters to indicate one with a low amplitude (less than 5 mm).

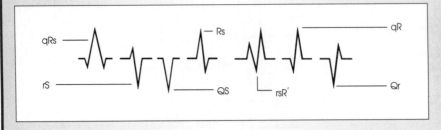

Whenever you're monitoring cardiac rhythm, remember that the waveform you see represents only the heart's electrical activity. It doesn't guarantee a mechanical contraction of the heart and a subsequent pulse. The contraction could be weak, as happens with premature ventricular contractions, or absent, as happens with pulseless electrical activity. So, before you treat what the strip shows, check the patient.

Pay special attention to the duration and configuration when evaluating a QRS complex. A normal complex has the following characteristics.

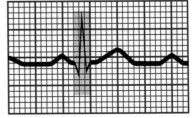

■ Location: follows the PR interval
■ Amplitude: 5 to 30 mm high, but differs for each lead used
■ Duration: 0.06 to 0.10 second or half of the PR interval (Duration is measured from the beginning of the Q wave to the end of the S wave or from the beginning of the R wave if the Q wave is absent.)
■ Configuration: consists of the Q wave (the first negative deflection, or deflection below the baseline, after the P wave), the R wave (the first positive deflection after the Q wave), and the S wave (the first negative deflection after the R wave) (You may not always see all three waves. It may also look different in each lead.) (See *QRS waveform variety.*)
■ Deflection: positive (with most of the complex above the baseline) in leads I, II, III, aV_L, aV_F, and V_4 to V_6, negative in leads aV_R and V_1 to V_2, and biphasic in lead V_3

Remember that the QRS complex represents intraventricular conduction time. That's why identifying and correctly interpreting it is so crucial. If no P wave appears with the QRS complex, then the impulse may have originated in the ventricles, indicating a ventricular arrhythmia.

Deep, wide Q waves may represent a myocardial infarction. In this case, the Q wave amplitude (depth) is greater than or equal to 25% of the

Changes in the ST segment

Closely monitoring the ST segment on a patient's electrocardiogram can help you detect myocardial ischemia or injury before infarction develops.

ST-SEGMENT DEPRESSION

An ST segment is considered depressed when it's 0.5 mm or more below the baseline. A depressed ST segment may indicate myocardial ischemia or digoxin toxicity.

ST-SEGMENT ELEVATION

An ST segment is considered elevated when it's 1 mm or more above the baseline. An elevated ST segment may indicate myocardial injury.

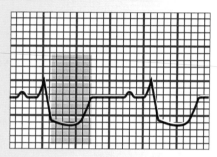
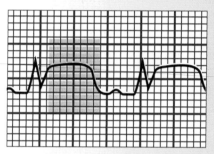

height of the succeeding R wave, or the duration of the Q wave is 0.04 second or more. A notched R wave may signify a bundle-branch block. A widened QRS complex (greater than 0.12 second) may signify a ventricular conduction delay. A missing QRS complex may indicate AV block or ventricular standstill.

ST SEGMENT

The ST segment represents the end of ventricular conduction or depolarization and the beginning of ventricular recovery or repolarization. The point that marks the end of the QRS complex and the beginning of the ST segment is known as the *J point.*

Pay special attention to the deflection of an ST segment. A normal ST segment has the following characteristics (amplitude, duration, and configuration aren't observed).

- Location: extends from the S wave to the beginning of the T wave
- Deflection: usually isoelectric or on the baseline (neither positive nor negative); may vary from –0.5 to +1 mm in some precordial leads

A change in the ST segment may indicate myocardial injury or ischemia. An ST segment may become either elevated or depressed. (See *Changes in the ST segment.*)

T WAVE

The peak of the T wave represents the relative refractory period of repolarization or ventricular recovery. When evaluating a T wave, look at the amplitude, configuration, and deflection.

Normal T waves have the following characteristics (duration isn't measured).

- Location: follows the ST segment
- Amplitude: 0.5 mm in leads I, II, and III and up to 10 mm in the precordial leads
- Configuration: typically rounded and smooth
- Deflection: usually positive or upright in leads I, II, and V_2 to V_6; inverted in lead aV_R; variable in leads III and V_1

The T wave's peak represents the relative refractory period of ventricular repolarization, a period during which cells are especially vulnerable to extra stimuli. Bumps in a T wave may indicate that a P wave is hidden in it. If a P wave is hidden, atrial depolarization has occurred, the impulse having originated at a site above the ventricles.

Tall, peaked, or "tented" T waves may indicate myocardial injury or electrolyte imbalances such as hyperkalemia. Inverted T waves in leads I, II, aV_L, aV_F, or V_2 through V_6 may represent myocardial ischemia. Heavily notched or pointed T waves in an adult may indicate pericarditis.

QT INTERVAL

The QT interval measures the time needed for ventricular depolarization and repolarization. The length of the QT interval varies according to heart rate. The faster the heart rate, the shorter the QT interval. When checking the QT interval, look closely at the duration.

A normal QT interval has the following characteristics (amplitude, configuration, and deflection aren't observed).

- Location: extends from the beginning of the QRS complex to the end of the T wave
- Duration: varies according to age, gender, and heart rate; usually lasts from 0.36 to 0.44 second; shouldn't be greater than half the distance between the two consecutive R waves (called the *R-R interval*) when the rhythm is regular

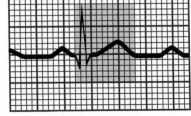

The QT interval measures the time needed for ventricular depolarization and repolarization. Prolonged QT intervals indicate that ventricular repolarization time is slowed, meaning that the relative refractory, or vulnerable, period of the cardiac cycle is longer.

This variation is also associated with certain medications, such as class I antiarrhythmics. Prolonged QT syndrome is a congenital conduction-system defect present in certain families. Short QT intervals may result from digoxin toxicity or electrolyte imbalances such as hypercalcemia.

U WAVE

The U wave represents repolarization of the His-Purkinje system or ventricular conduction fibers. It isn't present on every rhythm strip. The configuration is the most important characteristic of the U wave.

When present, a normal U wave has the following characteristics (amplitude and duration aren't measured).

- Location: follows the T wave
- Configuration: typically upright and rounded
- Deflection: upright

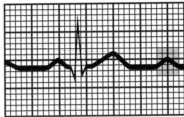

The U wave may not appear on an ECG. A prominent U wave may result from hypercalcemia, hypokalemia, or digoxin toxicity.

■ Normal sinus rhythm

Before you can recognize an arrhythmia, you first need to be able to recognize a normal cardiac rhythm. The term *arrhythmia* literally means an absence of rhythm. The more accurate term *dysrhythmia* means an abnormality in rhythm. These terms, however, are typically used interchangeably.

Normal sinus rhythm (NSR) occurs when an impulse starts in the sinus node and progresses to the ventricles through a normal conduction pathway — from the sinus node to the atria and AV node, through the bundle of His, to the bundle branches, and on to the Purkinje fibers. No premature or aberrant contractions are present. NSR is the standard against which all other rhythms are compared. (See *Recognizing normal sinus rhythm*, page 34.)

Practice the eight-step method, described below, to analyze an ECG strip with a normal cardiac rhythm, known as *NSR*. The ECG characteristics of NSR include:

- Rhythm — atrial and ventricular rhythms are regular
- Rate — atrial and ventricular rates are 60 to 100 beats/minute, the SA node's normal firing rate
- P wave — normally shaped (round and smooth) and upright in lead II; all P waves similar in size and shape; one P wave for every QRS complex
- PR interval — within normal limits (0.12 to 0.20 second)
- QRS complex — within normal limits (0.06 to 0.10 second)
- T wave — normally shaped; upright and rounded in lead II

Recognizing normal sinus rhythm

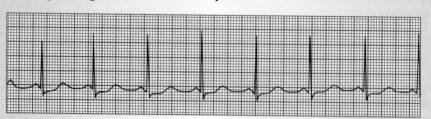

Rhythm
- Atrial regular
- Ventricular regular

Rate
- 60 to 100 beats/minute (sinoatrial node's normal firing rate)

P wave
- Normal shape (round and smooth)
- Upright in lead II
- One for every QRS complex
- All similar in size and shape

PR interval
- Within normal limits (0.12 to 0.20 second)

QRS complex
- Within normal limits (0.06 to 0.10 second)

T wave
- Normal shape
- Upright and rounded in lead II

QT interval
- Within normal limits (0.36 to 0.44 second)

Other
- No ectopic or aberrant beats

- QT interval — within normal limits (0.36 to 0.44 second)
- Other — no ectopic or aberrant beats.

■ *The eight-step method*

Analyzing a rhythm strip is a skill developed through practice. You can use several methods, as long as you're consistent. Rhythm strip analysis requires a sequential and systematic approach such as the eight steps outlined here.

STEP 1: DETERMINE RHYTHM

To determine the heart's atrial and ventricular rhythms, use either the paper-and-pencil method or the caliper method. (See *Methods of measuring rhythm.*)

For atrial rhythm, measure the P-P intervals — that is, the intervals between consecutive P waves. These intervals should occur regularly, with only small variations associated with respirations. Then compare the P-P intervals in several cycles. Consistently similar P-P intervals indicate regular atrial rhythm; dissimilar P-P intervals indicate irregular atrial rhythm.

Methods of measuring rhythm

You can use either of the following methods to determine atrial or ventricular rhythm.

Paper-and-pencil method

■ Place the electrocardiogram (ECG) strip on a flat surface.
■ Position the straight edge of a piece of paper along the strip's baseline.
■ Move the paper up slightly so the straight edge is near the peak of the R wave.
■ With a pencil, mark the paper at the R waves of two consecutive QRS complexes, as shown below. This distance is the R-R interval.
■ Move the paper across the strip lining up the two marks with succeeding R-R intervals. If the distance for each R-R interval is the same, the ventricular rhythm is regular. If the distance varies, the rhythm is irregular.
■ Use the same method to measure the distance between P waves (the P-P interval) and determine whether the atrial rhythm is regular or irregular.

Caliper method

■ With the ECG on a flat surface, place one point of the calipers on the peak of the first R wave of two consecutive QRS complexes.
■ Adjust the caliper legs so the other point is on the peak of the next R wave, as shown below. This distance is the R-R interval.
■ Pivot the first point of the calipers toward the third R wave, and note whether it falls on the peak of that wave.
■ Check succeeding R-R intervals in the same way. If they're all the same, the ventricular rhythm is regular. If they vary, the rhythm is irregular.
■ Using the same method, measure the P-P intervals to determine whether the atrial rhythm is regular or irregular.

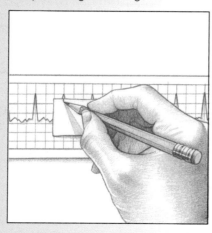

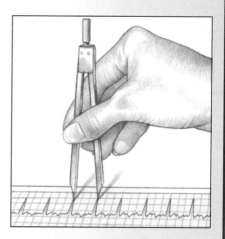

To determine the ventricular rhythm, measure the intervals between two consecutive R waves in the QRS complexes. If an R wave isn't present, use either the Q wave or the S wave of consecutive QRS complexes. The R-R intervals should occur regularly. Then compare R-R intervals in several cycles. As with atrial rhythms, consistently similar R-R intervals mean a regular ventricular rhythm; dissimilar R-R intervals point to an irregular ventricular rhythm.

After completing your measurements, ask yourself:
- Is the rhythm regular or irregular? Consider a rhythm with only slight variations, up to 0.04 second, to be regular.
- If the rhythm is irregular, is it slightly irregular or markedly so? Does the irregularity occur in a pattern (a regularly irregular pattern)?

STEP 2: CALCULATE RATE

You can use one of three methods to determine atrial and ventricular heart rates from an ECG waveform. Although these methods can provide accurate information, you shouldn't rely solely on them when assessing your patient. Keep in mind that the ECG waveform represents electrical, not mechanical, activity. Therefore, although an ECG can show you that ventricular depolarization has occurred, it doesn't mean that ventricular contraction has occurred. To determine this, you must assess the patient's pulse. So remember, always check a pulse to correlate it with the heart rate on the ECG.

- Times-10 method: The first method that's the simplest, quickest, and most common way to calculate rate is the times-10 method, especially if the rhythm is irregular. ECG paper is marked in increments of 3 seconds, or 15 large boxes. To calculate the atrial rate, obtain a 6-second strip, count the number of P waves on it, and multiply by 10. Ten 6-second strips equal 1 minute. Calculate ventricular rate the same way, using the R waves.
- 1,500 method: If the heart rhythm is regular, use the second method — the 1,500 method, so named because 1,500 small squares equals 1 minute. Count the number of small squares between identical points on two consecutive P waves, and then divide 1,500 by that number to get the atrial rate. To obtain the ventricular rate, use the same method with two consecutive R waves.
- Sequence method: The third method of estimating heart rate is the sequence method, which requires memorizing a sequence of numbers. For atrial rate, find a P wave that peaks on a heavy black line and assign the following numbers to the next six heavy black lines: 300, 150, 100, 75, 60, and 50. Then find the next P wave peak and estimate the atrial rate, based on the number assigned to the nearest heavy black line. Estimate the ventricular rate the same way, using the R wave. (See *Calculating heart rate.*)

STEP 3: EVALUATE P WAVE

When examining a rhythm strip for P waves, ask yourself:
- Are P waves present?
- Do the P waves have a normal configuration?
- Do all the P waves have a similar size and shape?
- Is there one P wave for every QRS complex?

STEP 4: DETERMINE PR-INTERVAL DURATION

To measure the PR interval, count the small squares between the start of the P wave and the start of the QRS complex; then multiply the number

Calculating heart rate

This table can help make the sequencing method of determining heart rate more precise. After counting the number of boxes between the R waves, use this table to find the rate.

For example, if you count 20 small blocks, or 4 large blocks, the rate would be 75 beats/minute. To calculate the atrial rate, use the same method with P waves instead of R waves.

Rapid estimation

This rapid-rate calculation is also called the *countdown method*. Using the number of large boxes between R waves or P waves as a guide, you can rapidly estimate ventricular or atrial rates by memorizing the sequence "300, 150, 100, 75, 60, 50."

Number of small blocks	Heart rate
5 (1 large block)	300
6	250
7	214
8	188
9	167
10 (2 large blocks)	150
11	136
12	125
13	115
14	107
15 (3 large blocks)	100
16	94
17	88
18	83
19	79
20 (4 large blocks)	75
21	71
22	68
23	65
24	63
25 (5 large blocks)	60
26	58
27	56
28	54
29	52
30 (6 large blocks)	50
31	48
32	47
33	45
34	44
35 (7 large blocks)	43
36	42
37	41
38	39
39	38
40 (8 large blocks)	37

of squares by 0.04 second. After performing this calculation, ask yourself:
- Does the duration of the PR interval fall within normal limits, 0.12 to 0.20 second (or 3 to 5 small squares)?
- Is the PR interval constant?

STEP 5: DETERMINE QRS-COMPLEX DURATION

When determining QRS-complex duration, make sure you measure straight across from the end of the PR interval to the end of the S wave, not just to the peak. Remember, the QRS complex has no horizontal components. To calculate duration, count the number of small squares between the beginning and end of the QRS complex and multiply this number by 0.04 second. Then ask yourself:

■ Does the duration of the QRS complex fall within normal limits, 0.06 to 0.10 second?

■ Are all QRS complexes the same size and shape? (If not, measure each one and describe them individually.)

■ Does a QRS complex appear after every P wave?

STEP 6: EVALUATE T WAVE

Examine the T waves on the ECG strip. Then ask yourself:

■ Are T waves present?

■ Do all of the T waves have a normal shape?

■ Could a P wave be hidden in a T wave?

■ Do all T waves have a normal amplitude?

■ Do the T waves have the same deflection as the QRS complexes?

STEP 7: DETERMINE QT-INTERVAL DURATION

Count the number of small squares between the beginning of the QRS complex and the end of the T wave, where the T wave returns to the baseline. Multiply this number by 0.04 second. Ask yourself:

■ Does the duration of the QT interval fall within normal limits, 0.36 to 0.44 second?

STEP 8: EVALUATE OTHER COMPONENTS

Note the presence of ectopic beats or other abnormalities such as aberrant conduction. Also, check the ST segment for abnormalities, and look for the presence of a U wave.

Now, interpret your findings by classifying the rhythm strip according to one or all of the following.

■ Origin of the rhythm: for example, sinus node, atria, AV node, or ventricles

■ Rate: normal (60 to 100 beats/minute), bradycardia (less than 60 beats/minute), or tachycardia (greater than 100 beats/minute)

■ Rhythm interpretation: normal or abnormal, for example, flutter, fibrillation, heart block, escape rhythm, or other arrhythmias

3 *Single-lead monitoring*

The two types of electrocardiogram (ECG) recordings are the 12-lead ECG and the single-lead ECG, commonly known as a *rhythm strip*. Both the 12-lead ECG and the rhythm strip obtained from the bedside cardiac monitor provide valuable information about heart function.

■ *Leadwire systems*

A three-, four-, or five-electrode system may be used for bedside cardiac monitoring. (See *Leadwire systems,* pages 40 and 41.) All three systems use a ground electrode to prevent accidental electrical shock to the patient.

A three-electrode system has one positive electrode, one negative electrode, and a ground. A four-electrode system has a right leg electrode that becomes a permanent ground for all leads. The popular five-electrode system is an extension of the four-electrode system and uses an additional exploratory chest lead to allow you to monitor any six modified chest leads as well as the standard limb leads. (See *Using a five-leadwire system,* page 42.) This system uses standardized chest placement. Wires that attach to the electrodes are usually color-coded to help you to place them correctly on the patient's chest.

Remember the needs of the patient when applying chest electrodes. For example, if defibrillation is anticipated, avoid placing the electrodes to the right of the sternum and under the left breast, where the paddles would be placed.

■ *Application of electrodes*

Before attaching electrodes to your patient, make sure he knows you're monitoring his heart rate and rhythm, not controlling them. Tell him not to become upset if he hears an alarm during the procedure; it probably just means a leadwire has come loose.

Explain the electrode placement procedure to the patient, provide privacy, and wash your hands. Expose the patient's chest and select elec-

Leadwire systems

The illustrations below show the correct electrode positions for some of the leads you'll use most often — the five-leadwire, three-leadwire, and telemetry systems. The abbreviations used are: RA for the right arm, LA for the left arm, RL for the right leg, LL for the left leg, C for the chest, and G for the ground.

Electrode positions
In the three- and five-leadwire systems, electrode positions for one lead may be identical to those for another lead. When that happens, change the lead selector switch to the setting that corresponds to the lead you want. In some cases, you'll need to reposition the electrodes.

Telemetry
In a telemetry monitoring system, you can create the same leads as the other systems with just two electrodes and a ground wire.

Five-leadwire system	**Three-leadwire system**	**Telemetry system**
LEAD I		
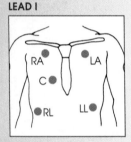	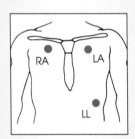	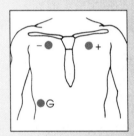
LEAD II		
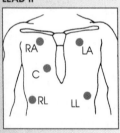	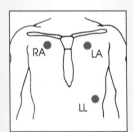	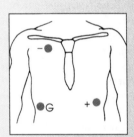
LEAD III		
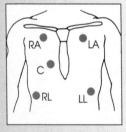	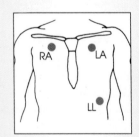	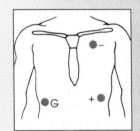

Leadwire systems *(continued)*

Five-leadwire system   Three-leadwire system   Telemetry system

LEAD MCL₁

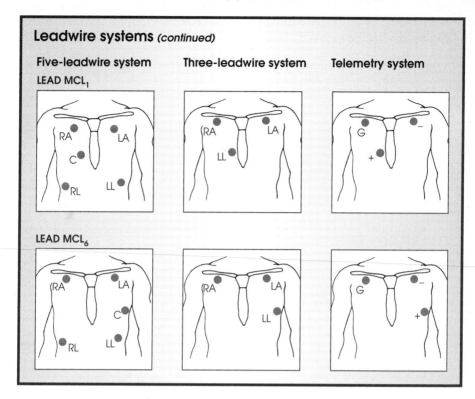

LEAD MCL₆

trode sites for the chosen lead. Choose sites over soft tissues or close to bone, not over bony prominences, thick muscles, or skin folds. Those areas can produce ECG artifact — waveforms not produced by the heart's electrical activity.

SKIN PREPARATION

Next, prepare the patient's skin. Use a special rough patch on the back of the electrode, a dry washcloth, or a gauze pad to briskly rub each site until the skin reddens. Be sure not to damage or break the skin. Brisk scrubbing helps to remove dead skin cells and improves electrical contact.

Hair may interfere with electrical contact; therefore, it may be necessary to clip areas with dense hair. Dry the areas if you moistened them. If the patient has oily skin, clean each site with an alcohol pad and allow it to air-dry. This process ensures proper adhesion and prevents alcohol from becoming trapped beneath the electrode, which can irritate the skin and cause skin breakdown.

APPLICATION OF ELECTRODE PADS

To apply the electrodes, remove the backing and make sure each pre-gelled electrode is still moist. If an electrode has become dry, discard it and select another. A dry electrode decreases electrical contact and interferes with waveforms.

Using a five-leadwire system

This illustration shows the correct placement of the leadwires for a five-leadwire system. The chest electrode shown is located in the lead V_1 position, but you can place it in any chest-lead position. The electrodes are color coded as follows.

- White — right arm (RA)
- Black — left arm (LA)
- Green — right leg (RL)
- Red — left leg (LL)
- Brown — chest (C)

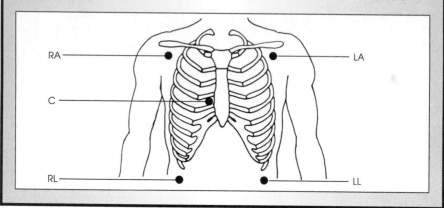

Apply one electrode to each prepared site using this method:
- Press one side of the electrode against the patient's skin, pull gently, and then press the opposite side of the electrode against the skin.
- Using two fingers, press the adhesive edge around the outside of the electrode to the patient's chest. This fixes the gel and stabilizes the electrode.
- Repeat this procedure for each electrode.
- Every 24 hours or according to your facility's policy and procedure, remove the electrodes, assess the patient's skin, and replace the old electrodes with new ones.

ATTACHING LEADWIRES

You'll also need to attach leadwires and the cable connections to the monitor. Then attach leadwires to the electrodes. Leadwires may clip on or, more commonly, snap on. If you're using the snap-on type, attach the electrode to the leadwire before applying it to the patient's chest. You can even do this step ahead of time if you know when the patient will arrive to prevent patient discomfort and disturbances of the contact between the electrode and the skin. When you use a clip-on leadwire, apply it after the electrode has been secured to the patient's skin. That way, applying the clip won't interfere with the electrode's contact with the skin.

■ *Observing cardiac rhythm*

After the electrodes are properly positioned, the monitor is on, and the necessary cables are attached, observe the screen. You should see the patient's ECG waveform. Although some monitoring systems allow you to make adjustments by touching the screen, most require you to manipulate knobs and buttons. If the waveform appears too large or too small, change the size by adjusting the gain control. If the waveform appears too high or too low on the screen, adjust the position dial.

Verify that the monitor detects each heartbeat by comparing the patient's apical rate with the rate displayed on the monitor. Set the upper and lower limits of the heart rate according to your facility's policy and the patient's condition. Heart rate alarms are generally set 10 to 20 beats/minute higher or lower than the patient's heart rate.

Monitors with arrhythmia detection generate a rhythm strip automatically whenever the alarm goes off. You can obtain other views of your patient's cardiac rhythm by selecting different leads. You can select leads with the lead selector button or switch.

To get a printout of the patient's cardiac rhythm, press the record control on the monitor. The ECG strip will be printed at the central console. Some systems print the rhythm from a recorder box on the monitor itself.

Most monitors can input the patient's name, date, and time as a permanent record; however, if the monitor you're using can't do this, label the rhythm strip with the patient's name, date, time, and rhythm interpretation. Add appropriate clinical information to the ECG strip, such as any medication administered, presence of chest pain, or patient activity at the time of the recording. Be sure to place the rhythm strip in the appropriate section of the patient's medical record.

■ *Troubleshooting monitor problems*

For optimal cardiac monitoring, you need to recognize problems that can interfere with obtaining a reliable ECG recording. (See *The look of monitor problems,* pages 44 and 45.) Causes of interference include artifact from patient movement and poorly placed or poorly functioning equipment.

An artifact, also called *waveform interference,* may be seen with excessive movement (somatic tremor). It causes the baseline of the ECG to appear wavy, bumpy, or tremulous. Dry electrodes may also cause this problem because of poor contact.

Electrical interference, also called *AC interference* or *60-cycle interference,* is caused by electrical power leakage. It may also result from interference from other room equipment or improperly grounded equipment. As a result, the lost current pulses at a rate of 60 cycles/second. This interference appears on the ECG as a baseline that's thick and unreadable.

The look of monitor problems

These illustrations present the most commonly encountered monitor problems, including the way to identify them, their possible causes, and interventions.

Waveform	Possible causes	Interventions
ARTIFACT (WAVEFORM INTERFERENCE) 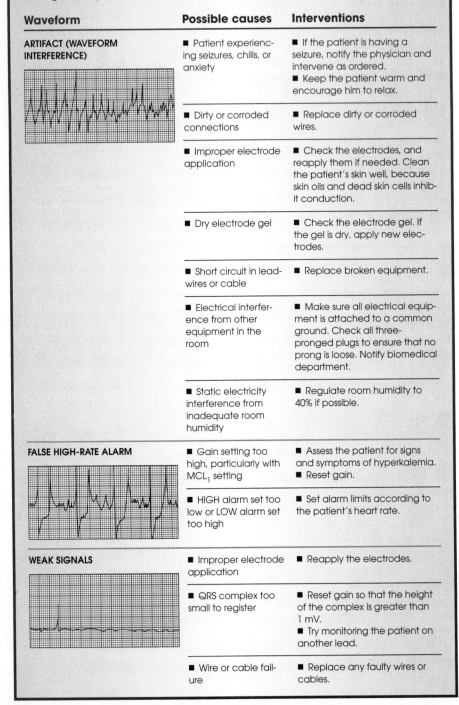	■ Patient experiencing seizures, chills, or anxiety	■ If the patient is having a seizure, notify the physician and intervene as ordered. ■ Keep the patient warm and encourage him to relax.
	■ Dirty or corroded connections	■ Replace dirty or corroded wires.
	■ Improper electrode application	■ Check the electrodes, and reapply them if needed. Clean the patient's skin well, because skin oils and dead skin cells inhibit conduction.
	■ Dry electrode gel	■ Check the electrode gel. If the gel is dry, apply new electrodes.
	■ Short circuit in lead-wires or cable	■ Replace broken equipment.
	■ Electrical interference from other equipment in the room	■ Make sure all electrical equipment is attached to a common ground. Check all three-pronged plugs to ensure that no prong is loose. Notify biomedical department.
	■ Static electricity interference from inadequate room humidity	■ Regulate room humidity to 40% if possible.
FALSE HIGH-RATE ALARM	■ Gain setting too high, particularly with MCL_1 setting	■ Assess the patient for signs and symptoms of hyperkalemia. ■ Reset gain.
	■ HIGH alarm set too low or LOW alarm set too high	■ Set alarm limits according to the patient's heart rate.
WEAK SIGNALS	■ Improper electrode application	■ Reapply the electrodes.
	■ QRS complex too small to register	■ Reset gain so that the height of the complex is greater than 1 mV. ■ Try monitoring the patient on another lead.
	■ Wire or cable failure	■ Replace any faulty wires or cables.

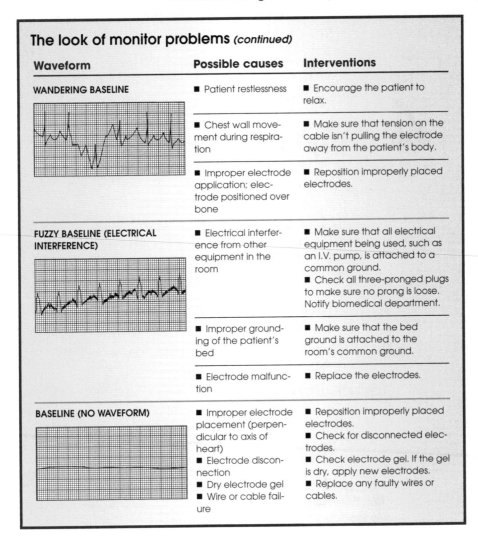

The look of monitor problems *(continued)*

Waveform	Possible causes	Interventions
WANDERING BASELINE	■ Patient restlessness	■ Encourage the patient to relax.
	■ Chest wall movement during respiration	■ Make sure that tension on the cable isn't pulling the electrode away from the patient's body.
	■ Improper electrode application; electrode positioned over bone	■ Reposition improperly placed electrodes.
FUZZY BASELINE (ELECTRICAL INTERFERENCE)	■ Electrical interference from other equipment in the room	■ Make sure that all electrical equipment being used, such as an I.V. pump, is attached to a common ground. ■ Check all three-pronged plugs to make sure no prong is loose. Notify biomedical department.
	■ Improper grounding of the patient's bed	■ Make sure that the bed ground is attached to the room's common ground.
	■ Electrode malfunction	■ Replace the electrodes.
BASELINE (NO WAVEFORM)	■ Improper electrode placement (perpendicular to axis of heart) ■ Electrode disconnection ■ Dry electrode gel ■ Wire or cable failure	■ Reposition improperly placed electrodes. ■ Check for disconnected electrodes. ■ Check electrode gel. If the gel is dry, apply new electrodes. ■ Replace any faulty wires or cables.

A wandering baseline undulates, meaning that all waveforms are present but the baseline isn't stationary. Movement of the chest wall during respiration, poor electrode placement, or poor electrode contact usually causes this problem.

Faulty equipment, such as broken leadwires and cables, can also cause monitoring problems. Excessively worn equipment can cause improper grounding, putting the patient at risk for accidental shock.

Be aware that some types of artifacts resemble arrhythmias and the monitor will interpret them as such. For example, the monitor may sense a small movement, such as the patient brushing his teeth, as a potentially lethal ventricular tachycardia. So, remember to treat the patient, not the monitor. The more familiar you become with your unit's monitoring system — and with your patient — the more quickly you can recognize and interpret monitor problems and act appropriately.

4 Arrhythmia recognition

Arrhythmias occur as a result of *abnormal impulse conduction* and may be classified based on the anatomic location of the electrical disturbance or classified according to rate. Bradycardia is a rate less than 60 beats/minute and tachycardia is a rate greater than 100 beats/minute.

■ Abnormal impulse conduction

Arrhythmias are thought to result from three mechanisms: altered automaticity, reentry, and afterdepolarization.

ALTERED AUTOMATICITY

The term *automaticity* refers to the ability of cardiac cells to initiate electrical impulses spontaneously. An increase in the automaticity of the atrial fibers can trigger abnormal impulses. Causes of increased automaticity include increased sympathetic stimulation, extracellular factors (such as hypoxia and digoxin toxicity), and conditions in which the function of the heart's normal pacemaker, the sinoatrial (SA) node, is diminished. For example, increased vagal tone or hypokalemia can increase the refractory period of the SA node and allow atrial fibers to initiate impulses.

REENTRY

In *reentry,* an impulse is delayed along a slow conduction pathway. Despite the delay, the impulse remains active enough to produce another impulse during myocardial repolarization. Reentry may occur with coronary artery disease, myocardial infarction (MI), or electrolyte imbalances and drugs.

AFTERDEPOLARIZATION

Afterdepolarization can occur as a result of cell injury, digoxin toxicity, and other conditions. An injured cell sometimes only partially repolarizes. Partial repolarization can lead to repetitive ectopic firing called *triggered activity*. The depolarization produced by triggered activity, known as afterdepolarization, can lead to atrial or ventricular tachycardia.

■ Anatomic location of electrical disturbance

Based on the location of the electrical disturbance, arrhythmias can be classified as sinus, atrial, junctional, and ventricular arrhythmias and atrioventricular (AV) blocks.

SINUS NODE ARRHYTHMIAS

When the heart functions normally, the SA node, also called the *sinus node*, acts as the primary pacemaker. The sinus node assumes this role because its automatic firing rate exceeds that of the heart's other pacemakers. In an adult at rest, the sinus node has an inherent firing rate of 60 to 100 times per minute. The autonomic nervous system (ANS) richly innervates the sinus node through the vagus nerve, a parasympathetic nerve, and several sympathetic nerves. Stimulation of the vagus nerve decreases the node's firing rate, and stimulation of the sympathetic system increases it. Sinus node arrhythmias result from changes in the automaticity of the sinus node, alterations in its blood supply, and ANS influences.

ATRIAL ARRHYTHMIAS

The most common cardiac rhythm disturbances, atrial arrhythmias result from impulses originating in the atrial tissue in areas outside the SA node. These arrhythmias can affect ventricular filling time and diminish atrial kick. The term *atrial kick* refers to the complete filling of the ventricles during atrial systole and normally contributes about 25% to ventricular end-diastolic volume.

JUNCTIONAL ARRHYTHMIAS

Junctional arrhythmias originate in the AV junction — the area in and around the AV node and the bundle of His. The specialized pacemaker cells in the AV junction take over as the heart's pacemaker if the SA node fails to function properly or if the electrical impulses originating in the SA node are blocked. These junctional pacemaker cells have an inherent firing rate of 40 to 60 beats/minute.

In normal impulse conduction, the AV node slows transmission of the impulse from the atria to the ventricles, which allows the ventricles to fill as much as possible before they contract. However, these impulses don't always follow the normal conduction pathway.

Because of the location of the AV junction within the conduction pathway, electrical impulses originating in this area cause abnormal depolarization of the heart. The impulse is conducted in a retrograde (backward) fashion to depolarize the atria and in an antegrade (forward) fashion to depolarize the ventricles.

Depolarization of the atria can precede depolarization of the ventricles, or the ventricles can be depolarized before the atria. Depolarization of the atria and ventricles can also occur simultaneously.

Retrograde depolarization of the atria results in inverted P waves in leads II, III, and aV_F, leads in which you would normally see upright P waves appear. An arrhythmia with an inverted P wave before the QRS complex and with a PR interval less than 0.12 second originates in the AV junction.

VENTRICULAR ARRHYTHMIAS

Ventricular arrhythmias originate in the ventricles below the bifurcation of the bundle of His. These arrhythmias occur when electrical impulses depolarize the myocardium using a different pathway from normal impulse conduction.

Ventricular arrhythmias appear on an electrocardiogram (ECG) in characteristic ways. The QRS complex in most of these arrhythmias is wider than normal because of the prolonged conduction time through — and abnormal depolarization of — the ventricles. The deflections of the T wave and the QRS complex are in opposite directions because ventricular repolarization as well as depolarization is abnormal. The P wave in many ventricular arrhythmias is absent because atrial depolarization doesn't occur.

When electrical impulses come from the ventricles instead of the atria, atrial kick is lost and cardiac output can decrease by as much as 30%. This decrease is one reason why patients with ventricular arrhythmias may show signs and symptoms of heart failure, including hypotension, angina, syncope, and respiratory distress.

Although ventricular arrhythmias may be benign, they're generally considered the most serious arrhythmias because the ventricles are ultimately responsible for cardiac output. Rapid recognition and treatment of ventricular arrhythmias increase the likelihood of successful resuscitation.

ATRIOVENTRICULAR BLOCK

AV heart block refers to an interruption or delay in the conduction of electrical impulses between the atria and the ventricles. The block can occur at the AV node (nodal), the bundle of His, or the bundle branches. When the site of the block is the bundle of His or the bundle branches the block is referred to as *infranodal AV block*. AV block can be partial (first or second degree) or complete (third degree).

The heart's electrical impulses normally originate in the SA node, so when those impulses are blocked at the AV node, atrial rates are usually normal (60 to 100 beats/minute). The clinical significance of the block depends on the number of impulses completely blocked and the resulting ventricular rate. A slow ventricular rate can decrease cardiac output and cause signs and symptoms, such as light-headedness, hypotension, and confusion.

AV blocks are traditionally classified in degrees: first-degree AV block; second-degree AV block, type I (Wenckebach or Mobitz I); second-degree AV block, type II (Mobitz II) AV block; and third-degree (complete) AV block.

◼ *Sinus arrhythmia*

In sinus arrhythmia, the rate usually stays within normal limits but the rhythm is irregular and corresponds to the respiratory cycle. Sinus arrhythmia can occur normally in athletes, children, and older adults, but it rarely occurs in infants. (See *Identifying sinus arrhythmia.*)

ASSESSMENT FINDINGS

The patient's peripheral pulse rate increases during inspiration and decreases during expiration. Sinus arrhythmia is easier to detect when the heart rate is slow; it may disappear when the heart rate increases, as with exercise.

If the arrhythmia is caused by an underlying condition, you may note signs and symptoms of that condition. Marked sinus arrhythmia may cause dizziness or syncope in some cases.

Identifying sinus arrhythmia

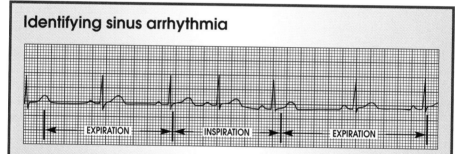

Rhythm
- Irregular
- Corresponds to the respiratory cycle
- P-P interval and R-R interval shorter during inspiration; longer during expiration
- Difference between the longest and the shortest P-P interval exceeds 0.12 second

Rate
- Usually within normal limits (60 to 100 beats/minute); rate may be less than 60 beats/minute
- Varies with respiration
- Increases during inspiration
- Decreases during expiration

P wave
- Normal size
- Normal configuration

PR interval
- May vary slightly
- Within normal limits

QRS complex
- Preceded by P wave
- Normal configuration

T wave
- Normal size
- Normal configuration

QT interval
- May vary slightly
- Usually within normal limits

Other
- Phasic slowing and quickening

INTERVENTIONS

Unless the patient is symptomatic, treatment usually isn't necessary. If sinus arrhythmia is unrelated to respirations, the underlying cause may require treatment.

When caring for a patient with sinus arrhythmia, observe the heart rhythm during respiration to determine whether the arrhythmia coincides with the respiratory cycle.

If sinus arrhythmia is drug induced (for example, from the use of morphine), the physician may decide whether to continue that drug therapy.

 RED FLAG If sinus arrhythmia develops suddenly in a patient taking digoxin, immediately notify the physician. The patient may be experiencing digoxin toxicity.

■ *Sinus bradycardia*

Sinus bradycardia is characterized by a sinus rate below 60 beats/minute and a regular rhythm. All impulses originate in the SA node. This arrhythmia's significance depends on its symptoms and underlying cause. Unless the patient shows symptoms of decreased cardiac output, no treatment is necessary. (See *Identifying sinus bradycardia.*)

ASSESSMENT FINDINGS

The patient will have a pulse rate of less than 60 beats/minute, with a regular rhythm. As long as he's able to compensate for the decreased cardiac output, he's likely to remain asymptomatic. If compensatory mecha-

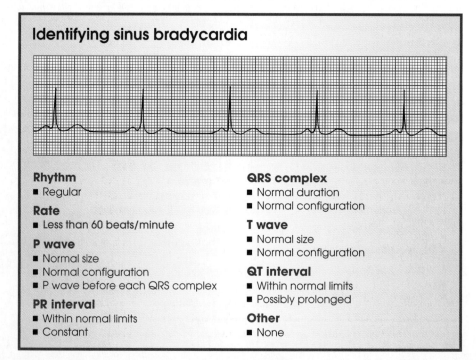

Identifying sinus bradycardia

Rhythm
- Regular

Rate
- Less than 60 beats/minute

P wave
- Normal size
- Normal configuration
- P wave before each QRS complex

PR interval
- Within normal limits
- Constant

QRS complex
- Normal duration
- Normal configuration

T wave
- Normal size
- Normal configuration

QT interval
- Within normal limits
- Possibly prolonged

Other
- None

nisms fail, however, signs and symptoms of declining cardiac output usually appear, including hypotension; cool, clammy skin; altered mental status; dizziness; blurred vision; crackles; dyspnea; and a third heart sound (S_3), indicating heart failure; chest pain; and syncope. Bradycardia-induced syncope (Stokes-Adams attack) may also occur.

INTERVENTIONS
If the patient is asymptomatic and his vital signs are stable, treatment generally isn't necessary. Continue to observe his heart rhythm, monitoring the progression and duration of the bradycardia. Evaluate his tolerance of the rhythm at rest and with activity. Review the medications he's taking. Check with the physician about stopping therapy with drugs that may be depressing the SA node, such as beta-adrenergic blockers, calcium channel blockers, or digoxin. Before giving these drugs, make sure the heart rate is within a safe range.

   If the patient is symptomatic, treatment aims to identify and correct the underlying cause. Meanwhile, the heart rate must be maintained with such drugs as atropine, dopamine, and epinephrine or with a transvenous or transcutaneous pacemaker. Keep in mind that a patient with a transplanted heart won't respond to atropine and may require pacing for emergency treatment. Treatment of chronic, symptomatic sinus bradycardia requires insertion of a permanent pacemaker.

■ Sinus tachycardia

Sinus tachycardia is an acceleration of the firing of the SA node beyond its normal discharge rate. Sinus tachycardia in an adult is characterized by a sinus rate of more than 100 beats/minute. The rate rarely exceeds 160 beats/minute, except during strenuous exercise; the maximum rate achievable with exercise decreases with age. (See *Identifying sinus tachycardia,* page 52.)

ASSESSMENT FINDINGS
The patient will have a pulse rate above 100 beats/minute, but with a regular rhythm. Usually, he'll be asymptomatic. However, if his cardiac output falls and compensatory mechanisms fail, he may experience hypotension, syncope, and blurred vision. He may report chest pain and palpitations, commonly described as a pounding chest or a sensation of skipped heartbeats. He may also report a sense of nervousness or anxiety. If heart failure develops, he may exhibit crackles, a third heart sound (S_3), and jugular vein distention.

INTERVENTIONS
Treatment usually isn't required unless the patient demonstrates signs and symptoms of decreased cardiac output or hemodynamic instability. If the patient is symptomatic, however, the focus of treatment is to maintain adequate cardiac output and tissue perfusion and to identify and correct the underlying cause. For example, if the tachycardia is caused by hemorrhage, treatment includes stopping the bleeding and replacing

Identifying sinus tachycardia

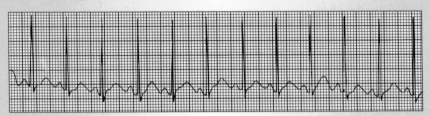

Rhythm
- Regular

Rate
- Greater than 100 beats/minute

P wave
- Normal size
- Normal configuration
- May increase in amplitude
- Precedes each QRS complex
- As heart rate increases, possibly superimposed on preceding T wave and difficult to identify

PR interval
- Within normal limits
- Constant

QRS complex
- Normal duration
- Normal configuration

T wave
- Normal size
- Normal configuration

QT interval
- Within normal limits
- Commonly shortened

Other
- None

blood and fluid losses. Keep in mind that tachycardia is typically the initial sign of pulmonary embolism. Maintain a high index of suspicion, especially if your patient has predisposing risk factors for thrombotic emboli.

 RED FLAG A sudden onset of sinus tachycardia after an MI may signal extension of the infarction. Prompt recognition is vital so that treatment can be started immediately.

If tachycardia leads to cardiac ischemia, treatment may include medications to slow the heart rate. The most commonly used drugs include beta-adrenergic blockers, such as atenolol and propranolol; and calcium channel blockers, such as diltiazem and verapamil.

Check the patient's drug history. Over-the-counter sympathomimetics, which mimic the effects of the sympathetic nervous system, may contribute to sinus tachycardia. Nose drops and cold formulas may contain sympathomimetics.

Also, question the patient about the use of alcohol, caffeine, and nicotine, each of which can trigger tachycardia. Advise him to avoid these substances. Ask about the use of illicit drugs, such as amphetamines and cocaine, which can also cause tachycardia.

Help to reduce fear and anxiety, which can aggravate the arrhythmia.

■ *Sinus arrest*

In sinus arrest, the normal sinus rhythm is interrupted by an occasional, prolonged failure of the SA node to initiate an impulse. Therefore, sinus arrest is caused by episodes of failure in the automaticity or impulse formation of the SA node. The atria aren't stimulated, and an entire PQRST complex is missing from the ECG strip. Except for this missing complex, or pause, the ECG usually remains normal. (See *Identifying sinus arrest.*)

ASSESSMENT FINDINGS

You won't be able to detect a pulse or heart sounds when sinus arrest occurs. Short pauses usually produce no symptoms. Recurrent or prolonged pauses may cause signs of decreased cardiac output, such as low blood pressure; altered mental status; cool, clammy skin; or syncope. The patient may also complain of dizziness or blurred vision.

INTERVENTIONS

An asymptomatic patient needs no treatment. If the patient is symptomatic, however, treatment focuses on the cause of the sinus arrest — for

Identifying sinus arrest

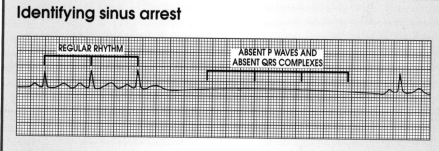

Rhythm
- Regular except during arrest (irregular as a result of missing complexes)

Rate
- Usually within normal limits (60 to 100 beats/minute) before arrest
- Length or frequency of pause may result in bradycardia

P wave
- Periodically absent, with entire PQRST complexes missing
- When present, normal size and configuration
- Precedes each QRS complex

PR interval
- Within normal limits when a P wave is present
- Constant when a P wave is present

QRS complex
- Normal duration
- Normal configuration
- Absent during arrest

T wave
- Normal size
- Normal configuration
- Absent during arrest

QT interval
- Within normal limits
- Absent during arrest

Other
- The pause isn't a multiple of the underlying P-P intervals

example, discontinuing drug therapy that affects SA node discharge or conduction, such as therapy with a beta-adrenergic blocker, a calcium channel blocker, and digoxin.

Examine the circumstances under which the pauses occur. If sinus arrest is recurrent, assess the patient for evidence of decreased cardiac output. Protect the patient from the risk of injury — for example, from a fall, which may result from syncope or near-syncopal episodes caused by a prolonged pause.

Document the patient's vital signs and the way he feels during pauses as well as the activities he was involved in at the time. Activities that increase vagal stimulation, such as Valsalva's maneuver or vomiting, increase the likelihood of sinus pauses.

Assess the patient for a progression of the arrhythmia. Notify the physician immediately if the patient's condition becomes unstable. If appropriate, be alert for signs of digoxin, quinidine, or procainamide toxicity. Obtain a serum digoxin level and a serum electrolyte level.

■ *Sinoatrial exit block*

In sinus exit block, the SA node discharges at regular intervals, but some impulses are delayed or blocked from reaching the atria, resulting in long sinus pauses. SA block results from failure to conduct impulses, whereas sinus arrest results from failure to form impulses in the SA node. In sinus exit block, the pause occurs for an indefinite period and ends with a sinus rhythm. (See *Identifying sinoatrial exit block.*)

ASSESSMENT FINDINGS
You won't be able to detect a pulse or heart sounds when sinus exit block occurs. Short pauses usually produce no symptoms. Recurrent or prolonged pauses may cause signs and symptoms of decreased cardiac output, such as low blood pressure; altered mental status; cool, clammy skin; and syncope. The patient may also complain of dizziness or blurred vision.

INTERVENTIONS
An asymptomatic patient needs no treatment. Treatment for symptomatic patients focuses on the cause of the sinus exit block. This may involve discontinuation of drug therapy that affects SA node discharge or conduction, such as therapy with a beta-adrenergic blocker, a calcium channel blocker, or digoxin.

Examine the circumstances under which the pauses occur. If the pauses are recurrent, assess the patient for evidence of decreased cardiac output. Protect the patient from the risk of injury, such as a fall, which may result from syncope or near-syncopal episodes caused by a prolonged pause.

Document the patient's vital signs and the way he feels during pauses as well as the activities he was involved in at the time. Activities that in-

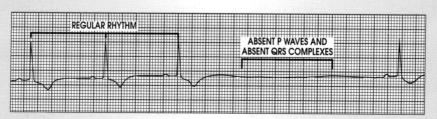

Identifying sinoatrial exit block

REGULAR RHYTHM

ABSENT P WAVES AND
ABSENT QRS COMPLEXES

Rhythm
■ Regular except during pause (irregular as result of pause)

Rate
■ Usually within normal limits (60 to 100 beats/minute) before pause
■ Length or frequency of pause may result in bradycardia

P wave
■ Periodically absent, with entire PQRST complexes missing
■ When present, normal size and configuration and precedes each QRS complex

PR interval
■ Within normal limits

■ Constant when a P wave is present

QRS complex
■ Normal duration
■ Normal configuration
■ Absent during a pause

T wave
■ Normal size
■ Normal configuration
■ Absent during a pause

QT interval
■ Within normal limits
■ Absent during a pause

Other
■ The pause is a multiple of the underlying P-P interval

crease vagal stimulation, such as Valsalva's maneuver or vomiting, increase the likelihood of sinus pauses.

Assess the patient for a progression of the arrhythmia. Notify the physician immediately if the patient's condition becomes unstable. If appropriate, be alert for signs of digoxin, quinidine, or procainamide toxicity. Obtain a serum digoxin level and a serum electrolyte level.

■ Sick sinus syndrome

Also known as *SA syndrome, sinus nodal dysfunction,* and *Stokes-Adams syndrome,* sick sinus syndrome (SSS) refers to a wide spectrum of SA node arrhythmias. SSS is caused by disturbances in the way impulses are generated or in the ability to conduct impulses to the atria. These disturbances either may be intrinsic or may be mediated by the ANS.

SSS usually shows up as bradycardia, with episodes of sinus arrest and SA block interspersed with sudden, brief periods of rapid atrial fibrillation. Patients are also prone to paroxysms of other atrial tachyarrhythmias, such as atrial flutter and ectopic atrial tachycardia, a condition sometimes referred to as *bradycardia-tachycardia* (or *"brady-tachy"*) *syndrome.*

Most patients with SSS are older than age 60, but anyone can develop the arrhythmia. It's rare in children, except after open-heart surgery that results in SA node damage. The arrhythmia affects men and women equally. The onset is progressive, insidious, and chronic. (See *Identifying sick sinus syndrome.*)

ASSESSMENT FINDINGS

The patient's pulse rate may be fast, slow, or normal, and the rhythm may be regular or irregular. You can usually detect an irregularity on the monitor or during palpation of the pulse, which may feel inappropriately slow, then rapid.

If you monitor the patient's heart rate during exercise or exertion, you may observe an inappropriate response to exercise, such as failure of the heart rate to increase. You may also detect episodes of brady-tachy syndrome, atrial flutter, atrial fibrillation, SA block, or sinus arrest on the monitor.

Other assessment findings depend on the patient's condition. For example, he may have crackles in the lungs, S_3, or a dilated and displaced left ventricular apical impulse if he has underlying cardiomyopathy. The

Identifying sick sinus syndrome

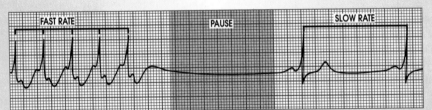

Rhythm
- Irregular with sinus pauses

Rate
- Fast, slow, or alternating
- Abrupt rate changes
- Interrupted by a long sinus pause

P wave
- Varies with rhythm changes
- May be normal size and configuration
- May be absent
- Usually precedes each QRS complex

PR interval
- Usually within normal limits
- Varies with rhythm changes

QRS complex
- Duration within normal limits
- Varies with rhythm changes
- Normal configuration

T wave
- Normal size
- Normal configuration

QT interval
- Usually within normal limits
- Varies with rhythm changes

Other
- Usually more than one arrhythmia on a 6-second strip

patient may also show signs and symptoms of decreased cardiac output, such as fatigue, hypotension, blurred vision, and syncope, a common experience with this arrhythmia. Syncopal episodes, when related to SSS, are referred to as *Stokes-Adams attacks.*

When caring for a patient with SSS, be alert for signs and symptoms of thromboembolism, especially if the patient has atrial fibrillation. Blood clots or mural thrombi forming in the heart can dislodge and travel through the bloodstream, resulting in decreased blood supply to the lungs, heart, brain, kidneys, intestines, or other organs. Assess the patient for neurologic changes such as confusion; vision disturbances; weakness; chest pain; dyspnea; tachypnea; tachycardia; and acute onset of pain. Early recognition allows for prompt treatment. Because an older adult with SSS may have an altered mental status, be sure to perform a thorough assessment to rule out such disorders as stroke, delirium, and dementia.

INTERVENTIONS

As with other sinus node arrhythmias, no treatment is generally necessary if the patient is asymptomatic. If the patient is symptomatic, however, treatment aims to alleviate signs and symptoms and correct the underlying cause of the arrhythmia.

Atropine or epinephrine may be given initially for symptom-producing bradycardia. A temporary pacemaker may be required until the underlying disorder resolves. Tachyarrhythmias may be treated with antiarrhythmic medications, such as digoxin and metoprolol. Unfortunately, medications used to suppress tachyarrhythmias may worsen underlying SA node disease and bradyarrhythmias. A permanent pacemaker may be necessary.

The patient may need an anticoagulant if he develops atrial fibrillation. The anticoagulant helps prevent thromboembolism and stroke, a complication of the condition.

When caring for a patient with SSS, monitor and document all arrhythmias as well as signs or symptoms experienced. Note changes in heart rate and rhythm related to changes in the patient's activity level.

Watch the patient carefully after starting a beta-adrenergic blocker, a calcium channel blocker, or other antiarrhythmic. If treatment includes anticoagulant therapy and pacemaker insertion, make sure the patient and his family receive appropriate instruction.

■ Premature atrial contractions

Premature atrial contractions (PACs) originate in the atria, outside the SA node. They arise from either a single ectopic focus or from multiple atrial foci that supersede the SA node as pacemaker for one or more beats. PACs are generally caused by enhanced automaticity in the atrial tissue. (See *Identifying premature atrial contractions,* page 58.)

Identifying premature atrial contractions

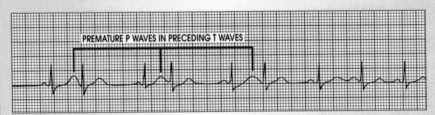

PREMATURE P WAVES IN PRECEDING T WAVES

Rhythm
- Atrial: Irregular
- Ventricular: Irregular
- Underlying: Possibly regular

Rate
- Atrial and ventricular: Vary with underlying rhythm

P wave
- Premature
- Abnormal configuration compared to a sinus P wave
- If varying configurations, multiple ectopic sites
- May be hidden in preceding T wave

PR interval
- Usually within normal limits
- May be shortened or slightly prolonged for the ectopic beat, depending on the origin of ectopic focus

QRS complex
- Conducted: Duration and configuration usually normal

- Nonconducted: No QRS complex follows premature atrial contraction (PAC)

T wave
- Usually normal
- May be distorted if P wave is hidden in T wave

QT interval
- Usually within normal limits

Other
- May be a single beat
- May be bigeminal (every other beat premature)
- May be trigeminal (every third beat premature)
- May be quadrigeminal (every fourth beat premature)
- May occur in couplets (pairs)
- Three or more PACs in a row indicate atrial tachycardia

PACs may be conducted or nonconducted (blocked) through the AV node and the rest of the heart, depending on the status of the AV and intraventricular conduction system. If the atrial ectopic pacemaker discharges too soon after the preceding QRS complex, the AV junction or bundle branches may still be refractory from conducting the previous electrical impulse. If they're still refractory, they may not be sufficiently repolarized to conduct the premature electrical impulse into the ventricles normally.

When a PAC is conducted, ventricular conduction is usually normal. Nonconducted, or blocked, PACs aren't followed by a QRS complex. At times, it may be difficult to distinguish nonconducted PACs from SA block. (See *Distinguishing nonconducted PACs from SA block.*)

ASSESSMENT FINDINGS

The patient may have an irregular peripheral or apical pulse rhythm when the PACs occur. Otherwise, the pulse rhythm and rate will reflect

LOOK-ALIKES

Distinguishing nonconducted PACs from SA block

To differentiate nonconducted premature atrial contractions (PACs) from sino-atrial (SA) block, check the following:
- Whenever you see a pause in a rhythm, look carefully for a nonconducted P wave, which may occur before, during, or just after the T wave preceding the pause.
- Compare T waves that precede a pause with the other T waves in the rhythm strip, and look for a distortion of the slope of the T wave or a difference in its height or shape. These are clues showing you where the nonconducted P wave may be hidden.
- If you find a P wave in the pause, check to see whether it's premature or if it occurs earlier than subsequent sinus P waves. If it's premature (see shaded area below, top), you can be certain it's a nonconducted PAC.
- If there's no P wave in the pause or T wave (see shaded area below, bottom), the rhythm is SA block.

NONCONDUCTED PAC

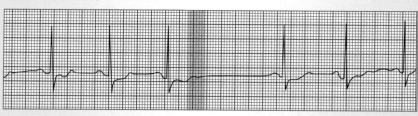

SA BLOCK

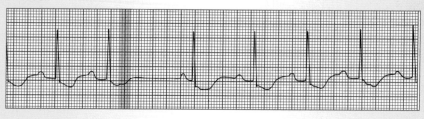

the underlying rhythm. Patients may complain of palpitations, skipped beats, or a fluttering sensation. In a patient with heart disease, signs and symptoms of decreased cardiac output, such as hypotension and syncope, may occur.

INTERVENTIONS

Most asymptomatic patients need no treatment. If the patient is symptomatic, however, treatment may focus on eliminating the cause, such as alcohol and caffeine. People with frequent PACs may be treated with drugs that prolong the refractory period of the atria. Such drugs include beta-adrenergic blockers and calcium channel blockers.

When caring for a patient with PACs, assess him to help determine factors that trigger ectopic beats. Tailor patient teaching to help the patient correct or avoid underlying causes. For example, the patient might need to avoid caffeine or learn stress reduction techniques to lessen anxiety.

If the patient has ischemic or valvular heart disease, monitor him for signs and symptoms of heart failure, electrolyte imbalance, and more severe atrial arrhythmias.

■ *Atrial tachycardia*

Atrial tachycardia is a supraventricular tachycardia, which means that the impulses driving the rapid rhythm originate above the ventricles. Atrial tachycardia has an atrial rate from 150 to 250 beats/minute. The rapid rate shortens diastole, resulting in a loss of atrial kick, reduced cardiac output, reduced coronary perfusion, and the potential for myocardial ischemia. (See *Identifying atrial tachycardia,* and *Distinguishing types of atrial tachycardia.*)

Identifying atrial tachycardia

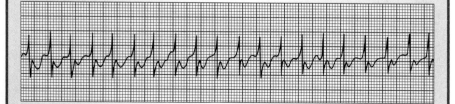

Rhythm
- Atrial: Usually regular
- Ventricular: Regular or irregular depending on atrioventricular (AV) conduction ratio and type of atrial tachycardia

Rate
- Atrial: Three or more consecutive ectopic atrial beats at 150 to 250 beats/minute; rarely exceeds 250 beats/minute
- Ventricular: Varies, depending on AV-conduction ratio

P wave
- Deviates from normal appearance
- May be hidden in preceding T wave
- If visible, usually upright and preceding each QRS complex

PR interval
- Within normal limits or may be difficult to measure if P wave can't be distinguished from preceding T wave

QRS complex
- Usually normal duration and configuration
- May be abnormal if impulses conducted abnormally through ventricles

T wave
- Usually visible
- May be distorted by P wave
- May be inverted if ischemia is present

QT interval
- Usually within normal limits
- May be shorter because of rapid rate

Other
- None

Distinguishing types of atrial tachycardia

Characteristics of atrial tachycardia with block:

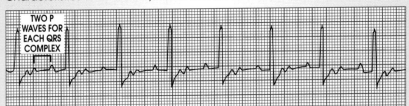

TWO P WAVES FOR EACH QRS COMPLEX

- *Rhythm:* atrial — regular; ventricular — regular if block is constant; irregular if block is variable
- *Rate:* atrial — 150 to 250 beats/minute and a multiple of ventricular rate; ventricular — varies with block
- *P wave:* abnormal
- *PR interval:* can vary but is usually constant for conducted P waves
- *QRS complex:* usually normal
- *T wave:* usually distorted
- *QT interval:* may be indiscernible
- *Other:* more than one P wave for each QRS complex

Characteristics of multifocal atrial tachycardia:

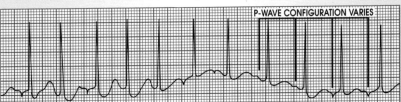

P-WAVE CONFIGURATION VARIES

- *Rhythm:* both irregular
- *Rate:* atrial — 100 to 250 beats/minute; ventricular — 100 to 250 beats/minute
- *P wave:* configuration varies; usually at least three different P-wave shapes must appear
- *PR interval:* varies
- *QRS complex:* usually normal, may become aberrant if arrhythmia persists
- *T wave:* usually distorted
- *QT interval:* may be indiscernible

Characteristics of paroxysmal atrial tachycardia:

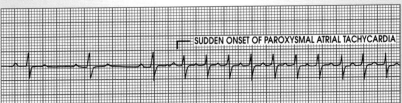

SUDDEN ONSET OF PAROXYSMAL ATRIAL TACHYCARDIA

- *Rhythm:* atrial and ventricular rhythms are regular
- *Rate:* 150 to 250 beats/minute
- *P wave:* abnormal; may not be visible or may be difficult to distinguish from the preceding T wave
- *PR interval:* usually within normal limits but may be unmeasurable if the P wave can't be distinguished from the preceding T wave
- *QRS complex:* usually normal, but can be aberrantly conducted
- *T wave:* usually distorted
- *QT interval:* may be indistinguishable
- *Other:* sudden onset, typically initiated by a premature atrial contraction

Three forms of atrial tachycardia are discussed here: atrial tachycardia with block, multifocal atrial tachycardia (MAT) or *chaotic atrial rhythm,* and paroxysmal atrial tachycardia (PAT). In MAT, the tachycardia originates from multiple foci. PAT is generally a transient event in which the tachycardia starts and stops suddenly.

ASSESSMENT FINDINGS

The patient with atrial tachycardia will have a rapid apical and peripheral pulse rate. The rhythm may be regular or irregular, depending on the type of atrial tachycardia. A patient with PAT may complain that his heart suddenly starts to beat faster or that he suddenly feels palpitations. Persistent tachycardia and rapid ventricular rate cause decreased cardiac output, resulting in hypotension and syncope.

INTERVENTIONS

Treatment depends on the type of tachycardia and the severity of the patient's symptoms. Because one of the most common causes of atrial tachycardia is digoxin toxicity, assess the patient who's taking digoxin for signs and symptoms of digoxin toxicity and monitor his blood digoxin level.

The Valsalva maneuver or carotid sinus massage may be used to treat PAT. These maneuvers increase parasympathetic tone, which results in a slowing of the heart rate. They also allow the SA node to resume function as the primary pacemaker.

Keep in mind that vagal stimulation can result in bradycardia, ventricular arrhythmias, and asystole. If vagal maneuvers are used, make sure resuscitative equipment is readily available.

Because carotid bruits may be absent, even with significant disease, carotid atherosclerosis might go undiagnosed in older adults. As a result, cardiac sinus massage shouldn't be performed in late middle-age and older patients. Embolic stroke may result if carotid massage is performed on a patient with significant atherosclerosis.

Drug therapy (pharmacologic cardioversion) may be used to treat atrial tachycardia. Appropriate drugs include adenosine, amiodarone, beta-adrenergic blockers, calcium channel blockers, and digoxin. When other treatments fail, or if the patient's condition is unstable, synchronized electrical cardioversion may be used.

In patients with chronic obstructive pulmonary disease (COPD), MAT is a common arrhythmia that commonly doesn't respond to antiarrhythmic therapy. Treatment is then directed at correcting hypoxia and electrolyte imbalance.

Atrial overdrive pacing (also called *rapid atrial pacing* or *overdrive suppression*) may also be used to stop the arrhythmia. This technique involves suppression of spontaneous depolarization of the ectopic pacemaker by a series of paced electrical impulses at a rate slightly higher than the intrinsic ectopic atrial rate.

 LEAD OF CHOICE Leads II, V_1, V_6 or MCL_1 or MCL_6 are the best choices for monitoring the patient with atrial tachycardia.

■ *Atrial flutter*

Atrial flutter, a supraventricular tachycardia, is characterized by a rapid atrial rate of 250 to 400 beats/minute, although the atrial rate is usually around 300 beats/minute. Originating in a single atrial focus, this rhythm results from a reentry mechanism and, possibly, increased automaticity.

On an ECG, the P waves lose their normal appearance because of the rapid atrial rate. The waves blend together in a sawtooth configuration called *flutter waves*, or *F waves*. These waves are the hallmark of atrial flutter. (See *Identifying atrial flutter.*)

Identifying atrial flutter

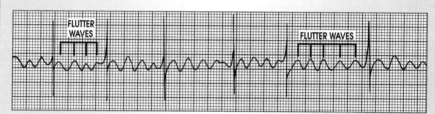

Rhythm
- Atrial: Regular
- Ventricular: Typically regular; may be irregular because cycles may alternate (depends on atrioventricular (AV) conduction pattern)

Rate
- Atrial: 250 to 400 beats/minute
- Ventricular: Usually 60 to 150 beats/minute (one-half to one-fourth of atrial rate) but varies depending on degree of AV block
- Usually expressed as a ratio (2:1 or 4:1, for example)
- Commonly 300 beats/minute atrial and 150 beats/minute ventricular, known as *2:1 block*
- Only every second, third, or fourth impulse is conducted to ventricles because the AV node usually won't accept more than 180 impulses/minute
- When atrial flutter is first recognized, ventricular rate typically exceeds 100 beats/minute

P wave
- Abnormal
- Sawtooth appearance known as *flutter waves or F waves*

PR interval
- Not measurable

QRS complex
- Duration: Usually within normal limits
- May be widened if flutter waves are buried within the complex

T wave
- Not identifiable

QT interval
- Not measurable because T wave isn't identifiable

Other
- Atrial rhythm may vary between a fibrillatory line and flutter waves (called *atrial fib-flutter*), with an irregular ventricular response
- May be difficult to differentiate atrial flutter from atrial fibrillation

ASSESSMENT FINDINGS

When caring for a patient with atrial flutter, you may note that the peripheral and apical pulses are normal in rate and rhythm. That's because the pulse reflects the number of ventricular contractions, not the number of atrial impulses.

If the ventricular rate is normal, the patient may be asymptomatic. If the ventricular rate is rapid, however, the patient may experience a feeling of palpitations. The loss of atrial kick from atrial flutter can result in a loss of 20% of normal end-diastolic volume. Combined with the decreased diastolic filling time associated with a rapid heart rate, the patient may exhibit signs and symptoms of reduced cardiac output.

INTERVENTIONS

The focus of treatment for patients with atrial flutter includes controlling the rate and converting the rhythm. Specific interventions depend on the patient's cardiac function, whether preexcitation syndromes are involved, and the duration (less than or greater than 48 hours) of the arrhythmia. For example, in atrial flutter with normal cardiac function and duration of rhythm less than 48 hours, electrical cardioversion may be considered; for duration greater than 48 hours, electrical cardioversion shouldn't be performed unless the patient is receiving anticoagulant therapy because of the increased risk of thromboembolism.

In patients with otherwise normal heart function, administer a beta-adrenergic blocker, such as metoprolol, or a calcium channel blocker, such as diltiazem, to control the ventricular rate.

In patients with impaired heart function (heart failure or ejection fraction less than 40%), use amiodarone, digoxin, or diltiazem to control ventricular rate. Be alert to the effects of digoxin, which depresses the SA node.

Recurrent atrial flutter may be treated with ablation therapy.

If electrical cardioversion is indicated, prepare the patient for I.V. administration of a sedative or an anesthetic as ordered. Keep resuscitative equipment at the bedside. Be alert for bradycardia because cardioversion can decrease the heart rate. Monitor the cardiac rhythm closely.

LEAD OF CHOICE Leads II and III are the best leads for monitoring the patient with atrial flutter.

The patient may develop an atrial rhythm that varies between a fibrillatory line and flutter waves. This variation is referred to as *atrial fibflutter*. The ventricular response is irregular. At times, it may be difficult to distinguish atrial flutter from atrial fibrillation. (See *Distinguishing atrial flutter from atrial fibrillation.*)

LOOK-ALIKES

Distinguishing atrial flutter from atrial fibrillation

It isn't uncommon to see atrial flutter that has an irregular pattern of impulse conduction to the ventricles. In some leads, this may be confused with atrial fibrillation. Here's how to tell the two arrhythmias apart.

Atrial flutter
- Look for characteristic abnormal P waves that produce a sawtooth appearance, referred to as *flutter waves,* or *F waves.* These can best be identified in leads II, III, and V_1 on the 12-lead electrocardiogram.
- Remember that the atrial rhythm is regular. You should be able to map the flutter waves across the rhythm strip. While some flutter waves may occur within the QRS or T waves, subsequent flutter waves will be visible and occur on time.

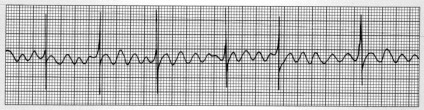

Atrial fibrillation
- Fibrillatory or *f waves* occur in an irregular pattern, making the atrial rhythm irregular.
- If you identify atrial activity that at times looks like flutter waves and seems to be regular for a short time, and in other places the rhythm strip contains fibrillatory waves, interpret the rhythm as atrial fibrillation. Coarse fibrillatory waves may intermittently look similar to the characteristic sawtooth appearance of flutter waves.

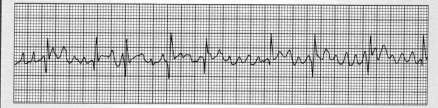

■ *Atrial fibrillation*

Atrial fibrillation, sometimes called *AFib,* is defined as chaotic, asynchronous, electrical activity in atrial tissue. It results from the firing of multiple impulses from numerous ectopic pacemakers in the atria. Atrial fibrillation is characterized by the absence of P waves and an irregularly irregular ventricular response.

When a number of ectopic sites in the atria initiate impulses, depolarization can't spread in an organized manner. Small sections of the atria are depolarized individually, resulting in the atrial muscle quivering instead of contracting. Uneven baseline fibrillatory waves — rather than clearly distinguishable P waves — appear on the ECG.

The AV node protects the ventricles from the 400 to 600 erratic atrial impulses that occur each minute by acting as a filter and blocking some of the impulses. The ventricles respond only to impulses conducted through the AV node, hence the characteristic, wide variation in R-R intervals. When the ventricular response rate drops below 100, atrial fibrillation is considered controlled. When the ventricular rate exceeds 100, atrial fibrilation is considered uncontrolled. (See *Identifying atrial fibrillation.*)

ASSESSMENT FINDINGS

When caring for a patient with atrial fibrillation, you may find that the radial pulse rate is slower than the apical rate. The weaker contractions that occur in atrial fibrillation don't produce a palpable peripheral pulse; only the stronger ones do.

The pulse rhythm will be irregularly irregular, with a normal or abnormal heart rate.

The loss of atrial kick from atrial fibrillation can result in a loss of 20% of normal end-diastolic volume; combined with the decreased dias-

Identifying atrial fibrillation

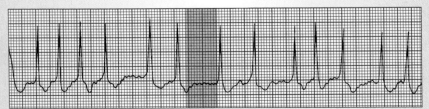

Rhythm
- Atrial: Irregularly irregular
- Ventricular: Irregularly irregular

Rate
- Atrial: Almost indiscernible, usually above 400 beats/minute; far exceeds ventricular rate because most impulses aren't conducted through the AV junction
- Ventricular: Usually 100 to 150 beats/minute but can be below 100 beats/minute

P wave
- Absent
- Replaced by baseline fibrillatory waves that represent atrial tetanization from rapid atrial depolarizations (see shaded area above)

PR interval
- Indiscernible

QRS complex
- Duration and configuration usually normal

T wave
- Indiscernible

QT interval
- Not measurable

Other
- Atrial rhythm may vary between fibrillatory line and flutter waves, called *atrial fib-flutter*
- It may be difficult to differentiate atrial fibrillation from atrial flutter and multifocal atrial tachycardia

tolic filling time associated with a rapid heart rate the patient may exhibit signs and symptoms of reduced cardiac output (such as hypotension and light-headedness). Patients with chronic atrial fibrillation may be able to compensate for the decreased cardiac output. Although these patients may be asymptomatic, they face a greater-than-normal risk of developing pulmonary, cerebral, or other thromboembolic events.

INTERVENTIONS

Treatment of atrial fibrillation aims to reduce the ventricular response rate to below 100 beats/minute. This reduction may be accomplished either by drugs that control the ventricular response or by a combination of electrical cardioversion and drug therapy, to convert the arrhythmia to normal sinus rhythm.

If the patient's condition is hemodynamically unstable, synchronized electrical cardioversion should be administered immediately. Electrical cardioversion is most successful if used within the first 48 hours after onset and less successful the longer the duration of the arrhythmia.

RED FLAG If atrial fibrillation has lasted longer than 48 hours, electrical cardioversion shouldn't be performed unless the patient is receiving anticoagulant therapy because of the risk of thromboembolism. If a thrombus forms in the atria, the resumption of normal contractions can result in systemic emboli.

Anticoagulant therapy is crucial in reducing the risk of thromboembolism. Heparin and warfarin are used for anticoagulation before and after cardioversion.

The focus of treatment with atrial fibrillation for patients whose conditions are hemodynamically stable includes controlling the rate, converting the rhythm, and providing anticoagulation if indicated. Specific interventions depend on the patient's cardiac function, whether preexcitation syndromes are involved, and the duration of the arrhythmia.

In patients with otherwise normal heart function, administer a beta-adrenergic blocker such as metoprolol, or a calcium channel blocker such as diltiazem, to control the rate.

In patients with impaired heart function (heart failure or ejection fraction less than 40%), use amiodarone, digoxin, or diltiazem to control the ventricular rate.

Symptomatic atrial fibrillation that doesn't respond to routine treatment may be treated with radiofrequency ablation therapy.

When assessing a patient with atrial fibrillation, assess the peripheral and apical pulses, and note the irregular pulse and differences in the radial and apical pulse rates (pulse deficit). Monitor cardiac rhythm closely.

LEAD OF CHOICE Lead II is the best choice for monitoring the patient with atrial fibrillation; however, you should be able to identify fibrillatory waves and the irregular R-R intervals in most leads.

Assess the patient for symptoms of decreased cardiac output and heart failure. If drug therapy is used, monitor serum drug levels and observe the patient for evidence of toxicity. Tell the patient to report pulse rate changes, syncope or dizziness, chest pain, and signs of heart failure, such as dyspnea and peripheral edema.

■ *Ashman's phenomenon*

Ashman's phenomenon refers to the aberrant conduction of premature supraventricular beats to the ventricles. (See *Identifying Ashman's phenomenon.*) This benign phenomenon is commonly associated with atrial fibrillation but can occur with any arrhythmia that affects the R-R interval.

ASSESSMENT FINDINGS
No signs and symptoms are related to this phenomenon.

INTERVENTIONS
No interventions are needed for this phenomenon, although they may be needed for accompanying arrhythmias.

Identifying Ashman's phenomenon

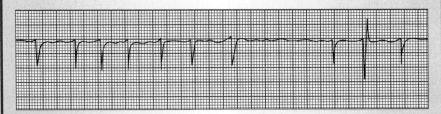

Rhythm
- Atrial: Irregular
- Ventricular: Irregular

Rate
- Reflects the underlying rhythm

P wave
- May be visible
- Abnormal configuration
- Unchanged if present in the underlying rhythm

PR interval
- Commonly changes on the premature beat, if measurable at all

QRS complex
- Altered configuration with right bundle-branch block (RBBB) pattern

T wave
- Deflection opposite that of QRS complex in most leads because of RBBB

QT interval
- Usually changed because of RBBB

Other
- No compensatory pause after an aberrant beat
- Aberrancy may continue for several beats and typically ends a short cycle preceded by a long cycle

■ *Wandering pacemaker*

Wandering pacemaker, also called *wandering atrial pacemaker,* is an atrial arrhythmia that results when the site of impulse formation shifts from the SA node to another area above the ventricles. The origin of the impulse may wander beat to beat from the SA node to ectopic sites in the atria or to the AV junctional tissue. The P wave and PR interval vary from beat to beat as the pacemaker site changes. (See *Identifying wandering pacemaker.*)

ASSESSMENT FINDINGS

Patients are generally asymptomatic and unaware of the arrhythmia. The pulse rate may be normal or below 60 beats/minute, and the rhythm may be regular or slightly irregular.

INTERVENTIONS

Usually, no treatment is needed for asymptomatic patients. If the patient is symptomatic, however, his medications should be reviewed and the

---

Identifying wandering pacemaker

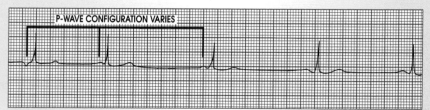

P-WAVE CONFIGURATION VARIES

Rhythm
- Atrial: Varies slightly, with an irregular P-P interval
- Ventricular: Varies slightly, with an irregular R-R interval

Rate
- Varies, but usually within normal limits or may be less than 60 beats/minute

P wave
- Altered size and configuration from changing pacemaker site with at least three different P-wave shapes visible
- May be absent or inverted or occur after QRS complex if impulse originates in the atrioventricular (AV) junction

PR interval
- Varies from beat to beat as pacemaker site changes

- Usually less than 0.20 second
- Less than 0.12 second if the impulse originates in the AV junction

QRS complex
- Duration and configuration usually normal because ventricular depolarization is normal

T wave
- Normal size and configuration

QT interval
- Usually within normal limits

Other
- May be difficult to differentiate wandering pacemaker from premature atrial contractions

LOOK-ALIKES

Distinguishing wandering pacemaker from PACs

Because premature atrial contractions (PACs) are commonly encountered, it's possible to mistake wandering pacemaker for PACs unless the rhythm strip is carefully examined. In such cases, you may find it helpful to look at a longer (greater than 6 seconds) rhythm strip.

Wandering pacemaker

■ Carefully examine the P waves. You must be able to identify at least three different shapes of P waves (see shaded areas below) in wandering pacemaker.
■ Atrial rhythm varies slightly, with an irregular P-P interval. Ventricular rhythm varies slightly, with an irregular R-R interval. These slight variations in rhythm result from the changing site of impulse formation.

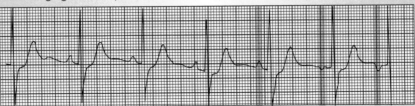

PAC

■ The PAC occurs earlier than the sinus P wave, with an abnormal configuration when compared with a sinus P wave (see shaded area below). It's possible, but rare, to see multifocal PACs, which originate from multiple ectopic pacemaker sites in the atria. In this setting, the P waves may have different shapes.
■ With the exception of the irregular atrial and ventricular rhythms as a result of the PAC, the underlying rhythm is usually regular.

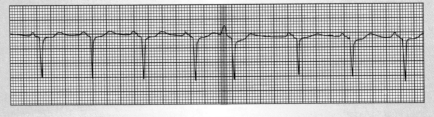

underlying cause investigated and treated. Assess the patient for signs of hemodynamic instability, such as hypotension and changes in mental status, and monitor the patient's heart rhythm. (See *Distinguishing wandering pacemaker from PACs.*)

■ *Premature junctional contractions*

A premature junctional contraction (PJC) is a junctional beat that occurs before a normal sinus beat; it interrupts the underlying rhythm and causes an irregular rhythm. These ectopic beats commonly occur as a re-

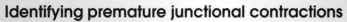

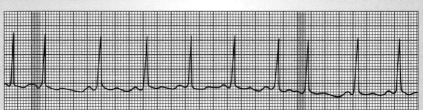

Identifying premature junctional contractions

Rhythm
- Atrial: Irregular during premature junctional contractions (PJCs)
- Ventricular: Irregular during PJCs
- Underlying rhythm possibly regular

Rate
- Atrial: Reflects underlying rhythm
- Ventricular: Reflects underlying rhythm

P wave
- Usually inverted (leads II, III, and aV$_F$) (see shaded area above)
- May occur before, during, or after QRS complex, depending on initial direction of depolarization
- May be hidden in QRS complex

PR interval
- Shortened (less than 0.12 second) if P wave precedes QRS complex
- Not measurable if no P wave precedes QRS complex

QRS complex
- Usually normal configuration and duration because ventricles usually depolarize normally

T wave
- Usually normal configuration

QT interval
- Usually within normal limits

Other
- Commonly accompanied by a compensatory pause reflecting retrograde atrial conduction

sult of enhanced automaticity in the junctional tissue or bundle of His. As with all impulses generated in the AV junction, the atria are depolarized in a retrograde fashion, causing an inverted P wave. The ventricles are depolarized normally. (See *Identifying premature junctional contractions.*)

ASSESSMENT FINDINGS
The patient is usually asymptomatic. He may complain of palpitations or a feeling of "skipped heart beats." You may be able to palpate an irregular pulse when PJCs occur. If PJCs are frequent enough, the patient may experience hypotension from a transient decrease in cardiac output.

INTERVENTIONS
PJCs don't usually require treatment unless the patient is symptomatic. In such patients, the underlying cause should be treated. For example, in digoxin toxicity, the medication should be discontinued and serum drug levels monitored.

Monitor the patient for hemodynamic instability as well. If ectopic beats occur frequently, the patient should decrease or eliminate triggers such as caffeine.

■ *Junctional rhythm*

A junctional rhythm, also referred to as *junctional escape rhythm,* is an arrhythmia originating in the AV junction. In this arrhythmia, the AV junction takes over as a secondary, or "escape," pacemaker. This takeover usually occurs only when the higher pacemaker site in the atria, the SA node, fails as the heart's dominant pacemaker.

Remember that the AV junction can take over as the heart's dominant pacemaker if the firing rate of the higher pacemaker sites falls below the AV junction's intrinsic firing rate, if the pacemaker fails to generate an impulse, or if the conduction of the impulses is blocked.

In a junctional rhythm, as in all junctional arrhythmias, the atria are depolarized by means of retrograde conduction. The P waves are inverted, and impulse conduction through the ventricles is normal. The normal intrinsic firing rate for cells in the AV junction is 40 to 60 beats/minute. (See *Identifying junctional rhythm.*)

Identifying junctional rhythm

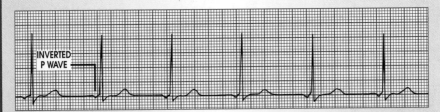

INVERTED P WAVE

Rhythm
- Atrial: Regular
- Ventricular: Regular

Rate
- Atrial: 40 to 60 beats/minute
- Ventricular: 40 to 60 beats/minute

P wave
- Usually inverted (leads II, III, and aV$_F$)
- May occur before, during, or after QRS complex
- May be hidden in QRS complex

PR interval
- Shortened (less than 0.12 second) if P wave precedes QRS complex

- Not measurable if no P wave precedes QRS complex

QRS complex
- Duration: Usually within normal limits
- Configuration: Usually normal

T wave
- Configuration: Usually normal

QT interval
- Usually within normal limits

Other
- Important to differentiate junctional rhythm from idioventricular rhythm (a life-threatening arrhythmia)

ASSESSMENT FINDINGS

A patient with a junctional rhythm will have a slow, regular pulse rate of 40 to 60 beats/minute. The patient may be asymptomatic. However, pulse rates under 60 beats/minute may lead to inadequate cardiac output, causing hypotension, syncope, or blurred vision.

INTERVENTIONS

Treatment for a junctional rhythm involves identification and correction of the underlying cause, whenever possible. If the patient is symptomatic, atropine may be used to increase the heart rate, or a temporary (transcutaneous or transvenous) or permanent pacemaker may be inserted.

 RED FLAG Because junctional rhythm can prevent ventricular standstill, it should never be suppressed.

Monitor the patient's serum digoxin and electrolyte levels, and watch for signs and symptoms of decreased cardiac output, such as hypotension, syncope, and blurred vision.

■ *Accelerated junctional rhythm*

An accelerated junctional rhythm is an arrhythmia that originates in the AV junction and is usually caused by enhanced automaticity of the AV junctional tissue. It's called *accelerated* because it occurs at a rate of 60 to 100 beats/minute, exceeding the inherent junctional escape rate of 40 to 60 beats/minute.

Because the rate is below 100 beats/minute, the arrhythmia isn't classified as junctional tachycardia. The atria are depolarized by means of retrograde conduction, and the ventricles are depolarized normally. (See *Identifying accelerated junctional rhythm*, page 74.)

ASSESSMENT FINDINGS

The pulse rate will be normal with a regular rhythm. The patient may be asymptomatic because accelerated junctional rhythm has the same rate as sinus rhythm. However, if cardiac output is decreased, the patient may exhibit signs and symptoms, such as hypotension, changes in mental status, and weak peripheral pulses.

INTERVENTIONS

Treatment for accelerated junctional rhythm involves identifying and correcting the underlying cause. Assessing the patient for signs and symptoms related to decreased cardiac output and hemodynamic instability is key, as is monitoring serum digoxin and electrolyte levels.

Identifying accelerated junctional rhythm

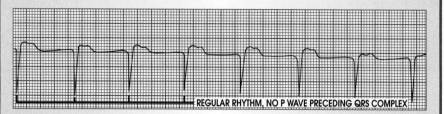

REGULAR RHYTHM, NO P WAVE PRECEDING QRS COMPLEX

Rhythm
- Atrial: Regular
- Ventricular: Regular

Rate
- Atrial: 60 to 100 beats/minute
- Ventricular: 60 to 100 beats/minute

P wave
- If present, inverted in leads II, III, and aV$_F$
- May occur before, during, or after QRS complex
- May be hidden in QRS complex

PR interval
- Shortened (less than 0.12 second) if P wave precedes QRS complex
- Not measurable if no P wave precedes QRS complex

QRS complex
- Duration: Usually within normal limits
- Configuration: Usually normal

T wave
- Usually within normal limits

QT interval
- Usually within normal limits

Other
- Important to differentiate accelerated junctional rhythm from accelerated idioventricular rhythm (a possibly life-threatening arrhythmia)

■ *Junctional tachycardia*

In junctional tachycardia, three or more PJCs occur in a row. This non-paroxysmal form of the arrhythmia has a gradual onset. It occurs as a result of enhanced automaticity of the AV junction, which causes the AV junction to override the SA node as the dominant pacemaker.

In junctional tachycardia, the atria are depolarized by retrograde conduction. Conduction through the ventricles is normal. (See *Identifying junctional tachycardia.*)

ASSESSMENT FINDINGS
The patient's pulse rate will be above 100 beats/minute and have a regular rhythm. Patients with a rapid heart rate may experience signs and symptoms of decreased cardiac output and hemodynamic instability, including hypotension.

INTERVENTIONS
The underlying cause should be identified and treated. If the cause is digoxin toxicity, the drug should be discontinued. In some cases of

Identifying junctional tachycardia

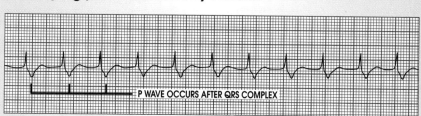

P WAVE OCCURS AFTER QRS COMPLEX

Rhythm
- Atrial: Usually regular but may be difficult to determine if P wave is hidden in QRS complex or preceding T wave
- Ventricular: Usually regular

Rate
- Atrial: Exceeds 100 beats/minute (usually 100 to 200 beats/minute) but may be difficult to determine if P wave is hidden in QRS complex
- Ventricular: Exceeds 100 beats/minute (usually 100 to 200 beats/minute)

P wave
- Usually inverted in leads II, III, and aV$_F$
- May occur before, during, or after QRS complex
- May be hidden in QRS complex

PR interval
- Shortened (less than 0.12 second) if P wave precedes QRS complex
- Not measurable if no P wave precedes QRS complex

QRS complex
- Duration: Within normal limits
- Configuration: Usually normal

T wave
- Configuration: Usually normal
- May be abnormal if P wave is hidden in T wave
- May be indiscernible because of fast rate

QT interval
- Usually within normal limits

Other
- May have gradual onset

digoxin toxicity, a digoxin-binding drug may be used to reduce the serum digoxin level. Patients with recurrent junctional tachycardia may be treated with ablation therapy, followed by permanent pacemaker insertion.

Monitor patients with junctional tachycardia for signs of decreased cardiac output. In addition, check digoxin and potassium levels and administer potassium supplements as ordered.

■ *Premature ventricular contractions*

Premature ventricular contractions (PVCs) are ectopic beats that originate in the ventricles and occur earlier than expected. PVCs may occur in healthy people without being clinically significant.

When PVCs occur in patients with underlying heart disease, however, they may herald the development of lethal ventricular arrhythmias, including ventricular tachycardia (VT) and ventricular fibrillation (VF).

Identifying premature ventricular contractions

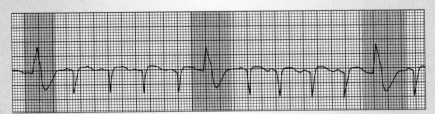

Rhythm
- Atrial: Irregular during premature ventricular contractions (PVCs)
- Ventricular: Irregular during PVCs
- Underlying rhythm may be regular

Rate
- Atrial: Reflects underlying rhythm
- Ventricular: Reflects underlying rhythm

P wave
- Usually absent in ectopic beat
- May appear after QRS complex with retrograde conduction to atria
- Usually normal if present in underlying rhythm

PR interval
- Not measurable except in underlying rhythm

QRS complex
- Occurs earlier than expected
- Duration: Exceeds 0.12 second
- Configuration: Bizarre and wide with PVC (see shaded areas)
- Usually normal in underlying rhythm

T wave
- Opposite direction to QRS complex

- May trigger more serious rhythm disturbances when PVC occurs on the downslope of the preceding normal T wave (R-on-T phenomenon)

QT interval
- Not usually measured except in underlying rhythm

Other
- PVC may be followed by full or occasionally an incomplete compensatory pause
- Full compensatory existing if the P-P interval encompassing the PVC has twice the duration of a normal sinus beat's P-P interval
- Incomplete compensatory existing if the P-P interval encompassing the PVC is less than twice the duration of a normal sinus beat's P-P interval
- Interpolated PVC: Occurs between two normally conducted QRS complexes without great disturbance to underlying rhythm
- Full compensatory pause absent with interpolated PVCs
- May be difficult to distinguish PVCs from aberrant ventricular conduction

PVCs may occur singly, in pairs (couplets), or in clusters. PVCs may also appear in patterns, such as bigeminy or trigeminy. (See *Identifying premature ventricular contractions*.)

In many cases, PVCs are followed by a compensatory pause. PVCs may be uniform in appearance, arising from a single ectopic ventricular pacemaker site, or multiform, originating from different sites or originating from a single pacemaker site but having QRS complexes that differ in size, shape, and direction.

PVCs may also be described as unifocal or multifocal. Unifocal PVCs originate from the same ventricular ectopic pacemaker site, whereas multifocal PVCs originate from different ectopic pacemaker sites in the ventricles.

ASSESSMENT FINDINGS

The patient experiencing PVCs usually has a normal pulse rate with a momentarily irregular pulse rhythm when a PVC occurs.

With PVCs, the patient will have a weaker pulse wave after the premature beat and a longer-than-normal pause between pulse waves. If the carotid pulse is visible, however, you may see a weaker arterial wave after the premature beat. When auscultating for heart sounds, you'll hear an abnormally early heart sound with each PVC.

A patient with PVCs may be asymptomatic; however, patients with frequent PVCs may complain of palpitations. The patient may also exhibit signs and symptoms of decreased cardiac output, including hypotension and syncope.

INTERVENTIONS

If the patient is asymptomatic, the arrhythmia probably won't require treatment. If symptoms or a dangerous form of PVCs occur, the type of treatment given will depend on the cause of the problem. Treatment is aimed at correcting the cause. For example, drug therapy may be adjusted or the patient's acidosis corrected. (See *Patterns of potentially dangerous PVCs,* page 78.)

If PVCs have a purely cardiac origin, drugs that suppress ventricular irritability (such as amiodarone, lidocaine, or procainamide) may be used.

Patients who have recently developed PVCs need prompt assessment, especially if they have underlying heart disease or complex medical problems. Patients with chronic PVCs should be closely observed for the development of more frequent PVCs or more dangerous PVC patterns.

Until effective treatment is begun, patients with PVCs accompanied by serious symptoms should have continuous ECG monitoring and ambulate only with assistance.

LEAD OF CHOICE Leads V_1, V_6, MCL_1, and MCL_6 are the best choices for identifying PVCs.

If, on discharge, the patient is taking an antiarrhythmic, family members should know how to contact the emergency medical system and perform cardiopulmonary resuscitation (**CPR**).

LIFE-THREATENING

Patterns of potentially dangerous PVCs

Some premature ventricular contractions (PVCs) are more dangerous than others. Here are examples of patterns of potentially dangerous PVCs.

Paired PVCs

Two PVCs in a row, called *paired PVCs* or a *ventricular couplet* (see shaded areas below), can produce ventricular tachycardia (VT). That's because the second contraction usually meets refractory tissue. A burst, or *salvo*, of three or more PVCs in a row is considered a run of VT.

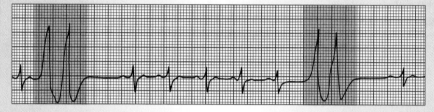

Multiform PVCs

Multiform PVCs, which look different from one another, arise from different sites or from the same site with abnormal conduction (see shaded areas below). Multiform PVCs may indicate severe heart disease or digoxin toxicity.

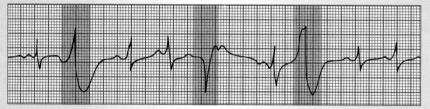

Bigeminy and trigeminy

PVCs that occur every other beat (*bigeminy*) or every third beat (*trigeminy*) may indicate increased ventricular irritability, which can result in VT or ventricular fibrillation (see shaded areas below). The rhythm strip shown below illustrates ventricular bigeminy.

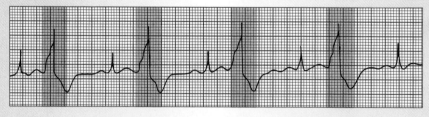

Patterns of potentially dangerous PVCs *(continued)*

R-on-T phenomenon
In R-on-T phenomenon, a PVC occurs so early that it falls on the T wave of the preceding beat (see shaded area below). Because the cells haven't fully repolarized, VT or ventricular fibrillation can result.

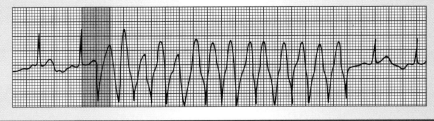

■ *Idioventricular rhythm*

Idioventricular rhythm, also referred to as *ventricular escape rhythm,* originates in an escape pacemaker site in the ventricles. The inherent firing rate of this ectopic pacemaker is usually 20 to 40 beats/minute. The rhythm acts as a safety mechanism by preventing ventricular standstill, or asystole — the absence of electrical activity in the ventricles. When fewer than three QRS complexes arising from the escape pacemaker occur, they're called *ventricular escape beats* or *complexes.* (See *Identifying idioventricular rhythm,* page 80.)

When the rate of an ectopic pacemaker site in the ventricles is less than 100 beats/minute but exceeds the inherent ventricular escape rate of 20 to 40 beats/minute, it's called *accelerated idioventricular rhythm* (AIVR). (See *Identifying accelerated idioventricular rhythm,* page 81.) The rate of AIVR isn't fast enough to be considered ventricular tachycardia. The rhythm is usually related to enhanced automaticity of the ventricular tissue. AIVR and idioventricular rhythm share the same ECG characteristics, differing only in heart rate.

ASSESSMENT FINDINGS
The patient with continuous idioventricular rhythm is generally symptomatic because of the marked reduction in cardiac output that occurs with the arrhythmia. The ventricular rhythm is usually regular at a rate of 20 to 40 beats/minute (the inherent rate of the ventricles). With AIVR, the ventricular rhythm is regular with a rate of 40 to 100 beats/minute.

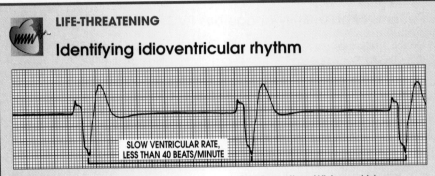

Identifying idioventricular rhythm

SLOW VENTRICULAR RATE, LESS THAN 40 BEATS/MINUTE

Rhythm
- Atrial: Usually can't be determined
- Ventricular: Usually regular

Rate
- Atrial: Usually can't be determined
- Ventricular: 20 to 40 beats/minute

P wave
- Usually absent

PR interval
- Not measurable because of absent P wave

QRS complex
- Duration: Exceeds 0.12 second because of abnormal ventricular depolarization

- Configuration: Wide and bizarre

T wave
- Abnormal
- Usually deflects in opposite direction from QRS complex

QT interval
- Usually prolonged

Other
- Commonly occurs with third-degree atrioventricular block
- If any P waves present, not associated with QRS complex

Blood pressure may be difficult to auscultate or palpate. The patient may experience dizziness, light-headedness, syncope, or loss of consciousness, especially with a heart rate of 40 beats/minute or less.

INTERVENTIONS

Treatment should be initiated immediately to increase the patient's heart rate, improve cardiac output, and establish a normal rhythm. Atropine may be administered to increase the heart rate.

If atropine isn't effective or if the patient develops hypotension or other signs of clinical instability, a pacemaker may be needed to reestablish a heart rate that provides enough cardiac output to perfuse organs properly. A transcutaneous pacemaker may be used in an emergency until a transvenous pacemaker can be inserted.

Identifying accelerated idioventricular rhythm

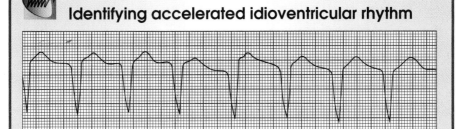

Rhythm
- Atrial: Can't be determined
- Ventricular: Usually regular

Rate
- Atrial: Usually can't be determined
- Ventricular: 40 to 100 beats/minute

P wave
- Usually absent

PR interval
- Not measurable

QRS complex
- Duration: Exceeds 0.12 second
- Configuration: Wide and bizarre

T wave
- Abnormal
- Usually deflects in opposite direction from QRS complex

QT interval
- Usually prolonged

Other
- If any P waves present, not associated with QRS complex

RED FLAG Remember that the goal of treatment doesn't include suppressing the idioventricular rhythm or AIVR because the rhythms act as a safety mechanism to protect the heart from ventricular standstill. They should never be treated with lidocaine or other antiarrhythmics that would suppress the escape beats.

Patients with idioventricular rhythm and AIVR need continuous ECG monitoring and constant assessment until treatment restores hemodynamic stability. Keep atropine and pacemaker equipment available at the bedside. Enforce bed rest until an effective heart rate has been maintained and the patient's condition is clinically stable. (See *Distinguishing AIVR from accelerated junctional rhythm,* page 82.)

Be sure to tell the patient and his family about the serious nature of this arrhythmia and the treatment it requires. If the patient needs a permanent pacemaker, teach the patient and his family how it works, how to recognize problems, when to contact the physician, and how pacemaker function will be monitored.

LOOK-ALIKES

Distinguishing AIVR from accelerated junctional rhythm

Accelerated idioventricular rhythm (AIVR) and accelerated junctional rhythm appear similar but have different causes. To distinguish between the two, closely examine the duration of the QRS complex and then look for P waves.

AIVR

- The QRS duration will be greater than 0.12 second.
- The QRS will have a wide and bizarre configuration.
- P waves are usually absent.
- The ventricular rate is generally between 40 and 100 beats/minute.

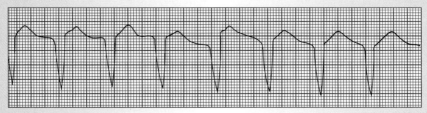

Accelerated junctional rhythm

- The QRS duration and configuration are usually normal.
- Inverted P waves generally occur before or after the QRS complex. However, remember that the P waves may also appear absent when hidden within the QRS complex.
- The ventricular rate is typically between 60 and 100 beats/minute.

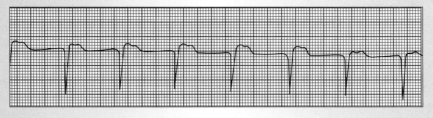

■ *Ventricular tachycardia*

Ventricular tachycardia (VT), also called *V-tach,* occurs when three or more PVCs strike in a row and the ventricular rate exceeds 100 beats/minute. This life-threatening arrhythmia may precede ventricular fibrillation and sudden cardiac death.

VT is an extremely unstable rhythm and may be sustained or nonsustained. When it occurs in short, paroxysmal bursts lasting less than 30 seconds and causing few or no symptoms, it's called *nonsustained.* When the rhythm is sustained, however, it requires immediate treatment to

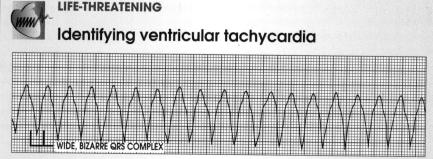

LIFE-THREATENING

Identifying ventricular tachycardia

WIDE, BIZARRE QRS COMPLEX

Rhythm
- Atrial: Can't be determined
- Ventricular: Usually regular but may be slightly irregular

Rate
- Atrial: Can't be determined
- Ventricular: Usually rapid (100 to 250 beats/minute)

P wave
- Usually absent
- If present, not associated with QRS complex

PR interval
- Not measurable

QRS complex
- Duration: Exceeds 0.12 second

- Configuration: Usually bizarre, with increased amplitude
- Uniform in monomorphic ventricular tachycardia (VT)
- Constantly changes shape in polymorphic VT

T wave
- If visible, occurs opposite the QRS complex

QT interval
- Not measurable

Other
- Ventricular flutter (VF): A variation of VT
- Torsades de pointes: A variation of polymorphic VT that's sometimes difficult to distinguish from VF

prevent death, even in patients initially able to maintain adequate cardiac output. (See *Identifying ventricular tachycardia.*)

ASSESSMENT FINDINGS

Although some patients have only minor symptoms initially, they still require rapid intervention to prevent cardiovascular collapse. Most patients with VT have weak or absent pulses. Low cardiac output will cause hypotension and a decreased level of consciousness (LOC), quickly leading to unresponsiveness if left untreated. VT may prompt angina, heart failure, or a substantial decrease in organ perfusion.

INTERVENTIONS

Treatment depends on the patient's clinical status. For example, is the patient conscious, does he have spontaneous respirations, and is a palpable carotid pulse present?

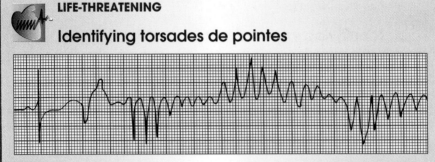

LIFE-THREATENING

Identifying torsades de pointes

Rhythm
- Atrial: Can't be determined
- Ventricular: May be regular or irregular

Rate
- Atrial: Can't be determined
- Ventricular: 150 to 300 beats/minute

P wave
- Not identifiable

PR interval
- Not measureable

QRS complex
- Usually wide

- Usually a phasic variation of electrical polarity, with complexes that point downward for several beats and then upward for several beats

T wave
- Not discernible

QT interval
- Prolonged

Other
- May be paroxysmal, starting and stopping suddenly

RED FLAG Patients with pulseless VT are treated the same as those with ventricular fibrillation and require immediate defibrillation. Treatment for patients with a detectable pulse depends on whether their condition is stable or unstable.

A patient whose condition is unstable will typically have a ventricular rate greater than 150 beats/minute and have serious signs and symptoms related to the tachycardia, which may include hypotension, shortness of breath, chest pain, or altered LOC. Such a patient is usually treated with immediate synchronized cardioversion.

A patient whose condition is clinically stable and who has VT and no signs of heart failure is treated differently. Treatment for such a patient is determined by whether the VT is monomorphic or polymorphic, whether the patient has normal or impaired cardiac function, and whether the baseline QT interval is normal or prolonged. Torsades de pointes is a form of polymorphic VT; when it occurs at an early age it's usually caused by congenital long QT syndrome. (See *Identifying torsades de pointes*. See also *Distinguishing ventricular flutter from torsades de pointes*.)

Patients with chronic, recurrent episodes of VT who are unresponsive to drug therapy may need an implanted cardioverter-defibrillator (ICD) to treat recurrent episodes of VT.

LOOK-ALIKES

Distinguishing ventricular flutter from torsades de pointes

Ventricular flutter, although rarely recognized, results from the rapid, regular, repetitive beating of the ventricles. It's produced by a single ventricular focus firing at a rapid rate of 250 to 350 beats/minute. The hallmark of this arrhythmia is its smooth sine-wave appearance.

Torsades de pointes is a variant form of ventricular tachycardia, with a rapid ventricular rate that varies between 150 and 300 beats/minute. It's characterized by QRS complexes that gradually change back and forth, with the amplitude of each successive complex gradually increasing and decreasing. This results in an overall outline of the rhythm commonly described as *spindle shaped.*

The illustrations shown here highlight key differences in the two arrhythmias.

Ventricular flutter
■ Smooth, sine-wave appearance

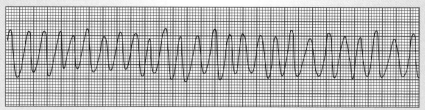

Torsades de pointes
■ Spindle-shaped appearance

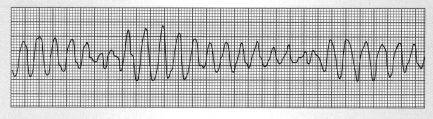

A 12-lead ECG and all other available clinical information are critical for establishing a specific diagnosis in a patient whose condition is stable and who has a wide QRS complex tachycardia of unknown type. If a definitive diagnosis of supraventricular tachycardia (SVT) or VT can't be established, the patient's treatment should be guided by whether cardiac function is preserved (ejection fraction greater than 40%).

Be sure to teach patients and their families about the serious nature of this arrhythmia and the need for prompt treatment. If your patient's condition is stable and he's undergoing electrical cardioversion, tell him that he'll be given a sedative, and possibly an analgesic, before the procedure.

If a patient will be discharged with an ICD or a prescription for a long-term antiarrhythmic, make sure that family members know how to contact the emergency medical system and perform CPR.

■ *Ventricular fibrillation*

Ventricular fibrillation, commonly called *V-fib*, is characterized by a chaotic, disorganized pattern of electrical activity. The pattern arises from electrical impulses coming from multiple ectopic pacemakers in the ventricles. (See *Identifying ventricular fibrillation*.)

ASSESSMENT FINDINGS

The patient in ventricular fibrillation is in full cardiac arrest, unresponsive, and without a detectable blood pressure or pulse. Whenever you see an ECG pattern resembling ventricular fibrillation, check the patient immediately and initiate definitive treatment.

INTERVENTIONS

When faced with a rhythm that appears to be ventricular fibrillation, always assess the patient first. Other events can mimic ventricular fibrillation on an ECG strip, including interference from an electric razor, shivering, or seizure activity.

RED FLAG Immediate defibrillation is the most effective treatment for ventricular fibrillation. CPR must be performed until the defibrillator arrives, to preserve the oxygen supply to the brain and other vital organs. Follow advanced cardiac life support guidelines and expect to give drugs, such as epinephrine and vasopressin. These drugs may be used for persistent ventricular fibrillation if the initial three attempts at electrical defibrillation fail to correct the arrhythmia. An antiarrhythmic, such as amiodarone or magnesium, may also be considered.

Automated external defibrillators (AEDs) are becoming more commonly used, especially in the out-of-facility setting, to provide early defibrillation. After a patient is confirmed to be unresponsive, breathless, and pulseless, the AED power is turned on and the electrode pads and cables attached. The AED can analyze the patient's cardiac rhythm and provide the caregiver with step-by-step instructions on how to proceed. These defibrillators can be used by people without medical experience as long as they're trained in the proper use of the device.

For the patient in ventricular fibrillation, successful resuscitation requires rapid recognition of the problem and prompt defibrillation. Many health care facilities and emergency medical systems have established protocols so that health care workers can initiate prompt treatment. Make sure that you know the location of your facility's emergency equipment and that you know how to use it.

You'll also need to teach the patient and his family how to use the emergency medical system after discharge from the facility. Family

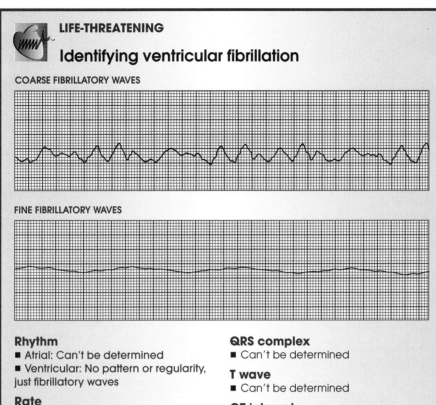

LIFE-THREATENING

Identifying ventricular fibrillation

COARSE FIBRILLATORY WAVES

FINE FIBRILLATORY WAVES

Rhythm
- Atrial: Can't be determined
- Ventricular: No pattern or regularity, just fibrillatory waves

Rate
- Atrial: Can't be determined
- Ventricular: Can't be determined

P wave
- Can't be determined

PR interval
- Can't be determined

QRS complex
- Can't be determined

T wave
- Can't be determined

QT interval
- Not measurable

Other
- Electrical defibrillation more successful with coarse fibrillatory waves than with fine waves, which indicate more advanced hypoxemia and acidosis

members may need instruction in CPR and in how to use the AED. Teach them about long-term therapies that help prevent recurrent episodes of ventricular fibrillation, including antiarrhythmic therapy and implantable cardioverter-defibrillators.

■ *Asystole*

Asystole, also called *ventricular asystole* and *ventricular standstill,* is the absence of discernible electrical activity in the ventricles. Although some electrical activity may be evident in the atria, these impulses aren't conducted to the ventricles. (See *Identifying asystole,* page 88.)

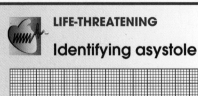

LIFE-THREATENING

Identifying asystole

Rhythm
- Atrial: Usually indiscernible
- Ventricular: Not present

Rate
- Atrial: Usually indiscernible
- Ventricular: Not present

P wave
- May be present

PR interval
- Not measurable

QRS complex
- Absent or occasional escape beats

T wave
- Absent

QT interval
- Not measurable

Other
- Looks like a nearly flat line on a rhythm strip except during chest compressions with cardiopulmonary resuscitation
- If the patient has a pacemaker, pacer spikes may show on the strip, but no P wave or QRS complex occurs in response

ASSESSMENT FINDINGS

The patient will be unresponsive and have no spontaneous respirations, discernible pulse, or blood pressure.

INTERVENTIONS

Immediate treatment for asystole includes effective CPR, supplemental oxygen, and advanced airway control with tracheal intubation. Resuscitation should be attempted unless evidence exists that these efforts shouldn't be initiated such as when a do-not-resuscitate order is in effect.

RED FLAG Remember to verify the presence of asystole by checking more than one ECG lead. Priority must also be given to searching for and treating identified potentially reversible causes, such as hypovolemia, cardiac tamponade, and tension pneumothorax. Early transcutaneous pacing may be considered, and I.V. epinephrine and atropine is administered, as ordered.

With persistent asystole (despite appropriate management), terminating resuscitation should be considered.

■ Pulseless electrical activity

Pulseless electrical activity, also known as *PEA*, is characterized by the presence of some type of electrical activity (which may be any rhythm)

LIFE-THREATENING

Identifying pulseless electrical activity

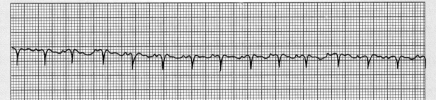

Rhythm
- Atrial: Same as underlying rhythm; becomes irregular as rate slows
- Ventricular: Same as underlying rhythm; becomes irregular as rate slows

Rate
- Atrial: Reflects underlying rhythm
- Ventricular: Reflects underlying rhythm; eventually decreases

P wave
- Same as underlying rhythm; gradually flattens and then disappears

PR interval
- Same as underlying rhythm; eventually disappears as P wave disappears

QRS complex
- Same as underlying rhythm; becomes progressively wider

T wave
- Same as underlying rhythm; eventually becomes indiscernible

QT interval
- Same as underlying rhythm; eventually becomes indiscernible

Other
- May be any rhythm; usually becomes a flat line indicating asystole within several minutes

without a detectable pulse. Although electrical depolarization occurs, no synchronous shortening of myocardial fibers does. As a result, no mechanical activity or contractions in the heart take place. (See *Identifying pulseless electrical activity*.)

ASSESSMENT FINDINGS

The patient will be unresponsive and have no spontaneous respirations, discernible pulse, or blood pressure.

INTERVENTIONS

Immediate treatment for pulseless electrical activity includes effective CPR, supplemental oxygen, and advanced airway control with tracheal intubation. Expect to give epinephrine and atropine according to advanced cardiac life support guidelines. Resuscitation should be attempted unless evidence exists that these efforts shouldn't be initiated such as when a do-not-resuscitate order is in effect.

Priority must also be given to searching for and treating identified potentially reversible causes. Treatment of reversible causes may include volume infusion for hypovolemia from hemorrhage, pericardiocentesis for cardiac tamponade, correction of electrolyte imbalances, needle decompression or chest tube insertion for tension pneumothorax, and surgery or thrombolytic therapy for massive pulmonary embolism.

RED FLAG It's important to remember that with PEA, there's electrical activity of the heart present without the presence of mechanical activity. As a result, any cardiac rhythm may be displayed on the monitor, but the patient won't have a pulse.

■ First-degree atrioventricular block

First-degree AV block occurs when there's a delay in the conduction of electrical impulses from the atria to the ventricles. This delay usually occurs at the level of the AV node, or bundle of His. First-degree AV block is characterized by a PR interval greater than 0.20 second. This interval remains constant beat to beat. Electrical impulses are conducted through the normal conduction pathway. However, conduction of these impulses takes longer than normal. (See *Identifying first-degree AV block*.)

ASSESSMENT FINDINGS
The patient's pulse rate will usually be normal and the rhythm regular. Most patients with first-degree AV block are asymptomatic because cardiac output isn't significantly affected. If the PR interval is extremely

---

Identifying first-degree AV block

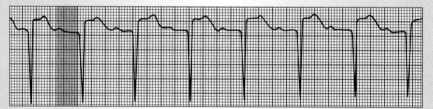

Rhythm
- Regular

Rate
- Within normal limits
- Atrial the same as ventricular

P wave
- Normal size
- Normal configuration
- Each followed by a QRS complex

PR interval
- Prolonged
- More than 0.20 second (see shaded area above)
- Constant

QRS complex
- Within normal limits (0.08 second) if conduction delay occurs in atrioventricular (AV) node
- If more than 0.12 second, conduction delay may be in His-Purkinje system

T wave
- Normal size
- Normal configuration
- May be abnormal if QRS complex is prolonged

QT interval
- Within normal limits

Other
- None

long, a longer interval between S_1 and S_2 may be noted on cardiac auscultation.

INTERVENTIONS

Treatment generally focuses on identification and correction of the underlying cause. For example, if a drug is causing the AV block, the dosage may be reduced or the drug discontinued. Close monitoring can help detect progression of first-degree AV block to a more serious form of block.

Evaluate a patient with first-degree AV block for underlying causes that can be corrected, such as drug therapy or myocardial ischemia. If the patient is prescribed a beta-adrenergic blocker, a calcium channel blocker, or digoxin, administer it cautiously and monitor the patient for ECG changes.

 RED FLAG Monitor the patient's rhythm closely. First-degree AV block may progress to a more severe type of AV block.

■ Type I second-degree atrioventricular block

Second-degree AV block occurs when some of the electrical impulses from the AV node are blocked and some are conducted through normal conduction pathways. Second-degree AV block is subdivided into type I second-degree AV block and type II second-degree AV block.

Type I second-degree AV block (also called *Wenckebach* or *Mobitz I block*) occurs when each successive impulse from the SA node is delayed slightly longer than the previous impulse. (See *Identifying type I second-degree AV block*, page 92.) This pattern of progressive prolongation of the PR interval continues until an impulse fails to be conducted to the ventricles (a P wave appears without a QRS complex).

Usually only a single impulse is blocked from reaching the ventricles, and after this nonconducted P wave or dropped beat, the pattern is repeated. This repetitive sequence of two or more consecutive beats followed by a dropped beat results in "group beating."

ASSESSMENT FINDINGS

The patient may be asymptomatic with type I second-degree AV block or may show signs and symptoms of decreased cardiac output, such as light-headedness or hypotension. Symptoms may be especially pronounced if the ventricular rate is slow.

INTERVENTIONS

Treatment may not be necessary if the patient is asymptomatic. A transcutaneous pacemaker may be required for a symptomatic patient until the arrhythmia resolves.

For a patient with serious signs and symptoms related to a low heart rate, atropine may be used to improve AV node conduction.

Identifying type I second-degree AV block

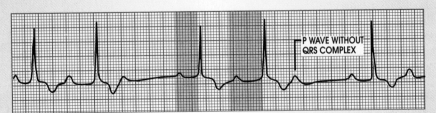

P WAVE WITHOUT QRS COMPLEX

Rhythm
- Atrial: Regular
- Ventricular: Irregular

Rate
- Atrial rate exceeds ventricular rate because of nonconducted beats
- Both rates usually within normal limits

P wave
- Normal size
- Normal configuration
- Each followed by a QRS complex except blocked P wave

PR interval
- Progressively longer (see shaded areas on strip) with each cycle until a P wave appears without a QRS complex
- Commonly described as "long, longer, dropped"
- Slight variation in delay from cycle to cycle

- After the nonconducted beat, shorter than the interval preceding it

QRS complex
- Usually within normal limits
- Periodically absent

T wave
- Normal size
- Normal configuration
- Deflection may be opposite that of the QRS complex

QT interval
- Usually within normal limits

Other
- Wenckebach pattern of grouped beats (footprints of Wenckebach)
- PR interval gets progressively longer and R-R interval shortens until a P wave appears without a QRS complex; cycle then repeats

RED FLAG Use atropine cautiously if the patient is diagnosed with an MI because atropine may worsen ischemia. Monitor all patients with type I AV block closely because the block may progress to a more severe form of AV block.

When caring for a patient with type I second-degree AV block, assess the patient's tolerance for the rhythm and the need for treatment to improve cardiac output. Evaluate the patient for possible causes of the block, including the use of certain drugs or the presence of myocardial ischemia.

Make sure the patient has a patent I.V. line. Provide patient teaching about a temporary pacemaker if indicated.

■ Type II second-degree atrioventricular block

Type II second-degree AV block (also known as *Mobitz II block*) is less common than type I, but more serious. It occurs when impulses from the SA node occasionally fail to conduct to the ventricles. This form of second-degree AV block occurs below the level of the AV node, either at the bundle of His, or more commonly at the bundle branches.

One of the hallmarks of this type of block is that, unlike type I second-degree AV block, the PR interval doesn't lengthen before a dropped beat and the PR interval is constant for conducted beats. (See *Identifying type II second-degree AV block.*) In addition, more than one nonconducted beat can occur in succession.

ASSESSMENT FINDINGS

Most patients who experience occasional dropped beats remain asymptomatic as long as cardiac output is maintained. As the number of dropped beats increases, the patient may experience signs and symptoms of decreased cardiac output, including fatigue, dyspnea, chest pain,

LIFE-THREATENING

Identifying type II second-degree AV block

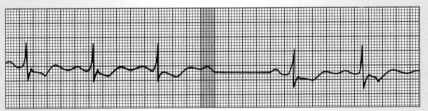

Rhythm
- Atrial: Regular
- Ventricular: Irregular
- Pauses correspond to dropped beat
- Irregular when block is intermittent or conduction ratio is variable
- Regular when conduction ratio is constant, such as 2:1 or 3:1

Rate
- Atrial exceeds ventricular
- Both may be within normal limits

P wave
- Normal size
- Normal configuration
- Some not followed by a QRS complex

PR interval
- Usually within normal limits but may be prolonged
- Constant for conducted beats

QRS complex
- Within normal limits or narrow if block occurs at bundle of His

- Widened and similar to bundle-branch block if block occurs at bundle branches
- Periodically absent

T wave
- Normal size
- Normal configuration

QT interval
- Within normal limits

Other
- PR and R-R intervals don't vary before a dropped beat (see shaded area above), so no warning occurs
- R-R interval that contains nonconducted P wave equals two normal R-R intervals
- Must be a complete block in one bundle branch and intermittent interruption in conduction in the other bundle for a dropped beat to occur

LOOK-ALIKES

Distinguishing nonconducted PACs from type II second-degree AV block

An isolated P wave that doesn't conduct through to the ventricle (P wave without a QRS complex following it; see shaded areas below) may occur with a nonconducted premature atrial contraction (PAC) or may indicate type II second-degree atrioventricular (AV) block. Mistakenly identifying AV block as nonconducted PACs may have serious consequences. The latter is generally benign; the former can be life-threatening.

Nonconducted PAC
If the P-P interval, including the extra P wave, isn't constant, it's a nonconducted PAC.

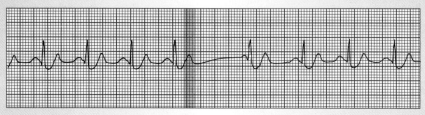

Type II second-degree AV block
If the P-P interval is constant, including the extra P wave, it's type II second-degree AV block.

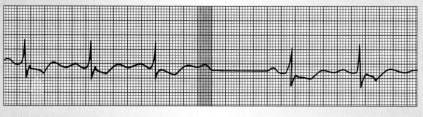

or light-headedness. On physical examination, you may note hypotension and a slow pulse, with a regular or irregular rhythm.

INTERVENTIONS

If the patient is experiencing serious signs and symptoms because of bradycardia, treatment goals include improving cardiac output by increasing the heart rate. Transcutaneous pacing should be initiated quickly when indicated, and I.V. dopamine infusion or I.V. epinephrine may be given to increase cardiac output. Type II second-degree AV block may also require placement of a permanent pacemaker. A transvenous pacemaker may be used until a permanent pacemaker can be inserted.

When caring for a patient with type II second-degree block, assess the patient's tolerance for the rhythm and the need for treatment to improve cardiac output. Evaluate for possible correctable causes, such as ischemia.

Keep the patient on bed rest, if indicated, to reduce myocardial oxygen demands. Administer oxygen therapy as ordered. Observe the patient's cardiac rhythm for progression to a more severe form of AV block or other arrhythmias. (See *Distinguishing nonconducted PACs from type II second-degree AV block.*) Teach the patient and his family about the use of pacemakers if the patient requires one.

■ *Third-degree atrioventricular block*

Also called *complete heart block,* third-degree AV block indicates the complete absence of impulse conduction between the atria and ventricles. In complete heart block, the atrial rate is generally faster than the ventricular rate. (See *Identifying third-degree AV block,* page 96.)

ASSESSMENT FINDINGS

Most patients with third-degree AV block experience significant signs and symptoms, including severe fatigue, dyspnea, chest pain, lightheadedness, changes in mental status, and changes in LOC. Hypotension, pallor, and diaphoresis may also occur. The peripheral pulse rate will be slow, but the rhythm will be regular.

A few patients will be relatively free from symptoms, complaining only that they can't tolerate exercise and that they're typically tired for no apparent reason. The severity of symptoms depends to a large extent on the resulting ventricular rate and the patient's ability to compensate for decreased cardiac output.

INTERVENTIONS

If the patient is experiencing serious signs and symptoms related to the low heart rate, or if the patient's condition seems to be deteriorating, transcutaneous pacing should be initiated quickly and I.V. dopamine infusion, or epinephrine may be given to increase cardiac output.

Asymptomatic patients with third-degree AV block should be prepared for insertion of a transvenous temporary pacemaker until a decision is made about the need for a permanent pacemaker. If symptoms develop, a transcutaneous pacemaker should be used until the transvenous pacemaker is placed.

Because third-degree AV block occurring at the infranodal level is usually associated with an extensive anterior-wall MI, patients are more likely to have permanent third-degree AV block, which most likely requires insertion of a permanent pacemaker.

Third-degree AV block occurring at the anatomic level of the AV node can result from increased parasympathetic tone associated with an inferior-wall MI. As a result, the block is more likely to be short lived. In these patients, the decision to insert a permanent pacemaker is commonly delayed to assess how well the conduction system recovers.

When caring for a patient with third-degree heart block, immediately assess the patient's tolerance of the rhythm and the need for interven-

LIFE-THREATENING

Identifying third-degree AV block

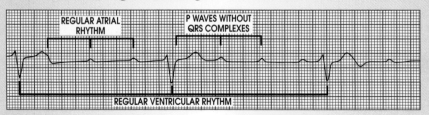

REGULAR ATRIAL RHYTHM

P WAVES WITHOUT QRS COMPLEXES

REGULAR VENTRICULAR RHYTHM

Rhythm
- Atrial: Regular
- Ventricular: Regular

Rate
- Atrial: 60 to 100 beats/minute (atria act independently under control of sinoatrial node)
- Ventricular: Usually 40 to 60 beats/minute in an intranodal block (a junctional escape rhythm)
- Ventricular: Usually less than 40 beats/minute in infranodal block (a ventricular escape rhythm)

P wave
- Normal size
- Normal configuration
- May be buried in QRS complex or T wave

PR interval
- Not measurable

QRS complex
- Configuration depends on location of escape mechanism and origin of ventricular depolarization
- Appears normal if the block is at the level of the atrioventricular (AV) node or bundle of His
- Widened if the block is at the level of the bundle branches

T wave
- Normal size
- Normal configuration
- May be abnormal if QRS complex originates in ventricle

QT interval
- Within normal limits

Other
- Atria and ventricles are depolarized from different pacemaker sites and beat independently of each other
- P waves occur without QRS complexes

tions to support cardiac output and relieve symptoms. Make sure that the patient has a patent I.V. line. Administer oxygen therapy as ordered. Evaluate the patient for possible correctable causes of the arrhythmia, such as drug therapy or myocardial ischemia. Minimize the patient's activity and maintain bed rest.

RED FLAG Atropine isn't indicated for third-degree AV block and wide QRS complexes or for Mobitz type II second-degree AV block. In such cases, atropine may increase the atrial rate, causing an increased AV nodal block. In patients with an acute MI, atropine can worsen ischemia and induce VT or ventricular fibrillation.

Part III
Interpreting
12-lead ECGs

5 Normal 12-lead ECG

The 12-lead electrocardiogram (ECG) is a diagnostic test that helps identify pathologic conditions, especially ischemia and acute myocardial infarction (MI). It provides a more complete view of the heart's electrical activity than a rhythm strip does and can be used to assess left ventricular function more effectively. Patients with conditions that affect the heart's electrical system may also benefit from a 12-lead ECG, including those with:

- cardiac arrhythmias
- heart chamber enlargement or hypertrophy
- digoxin or other drug toxicity
- electrolyte imbalances
- pulmonary embolism
- pericarditis
- pacemakers
- hypothermia.

Like other diagnostic tests, a 12-lead ECG must be viewed in conjunction with other clinical data. Therefore, always correlate the patient's ECG results with the history, physical assessment findings, and results of laboratory and other diagnostic studies as well as the drug regimen.

Remember, too, that an ECG can be done in various ways, including over a telephone line. (See *Transtelephonic cardiac monitoring.*) In fact, transtelephonic monitoring has become increasingly important as a tool for assessing patients at home and in other nonclinical settings.

The 12-lead ECG records the heart's electrical activity using a series of electrodes placed on the patient's extremities and chest wall. The 12 leads include three bipolar limb leads (I, II, and III), three unipolar augmented limb leads (aV_R, aV_L, and aV_F), and six unipolar precordial, or chest, leads (V_1, V_2, V_3, V_4, V_5, and V_6). These leads provide 12 different views of the heart's electrical activity. (See *Viewing ECG leads,* page 100.)

Scanning up, down, and across, each lead transmits information about a different area of the heart. The waveforms obtained from each lead vary depending on the lead's location in relation to the wave of depolarization passing through the myocardium.

Transtelephonic cardiac monitoring

Using a special recorder-transmitter, patients at home can transmit electrocardiograms (ECGs) by telephone to a central monitoring center for immediate interpretation. This technique, called *transtelephonic cardiac monitoring* (TTM), reduces health care costs and is now being used more often.

Nurses play an important role in TTM. Besides performing extensive patient and family teaching, they may operate the central monitoring center and help interpret ECGs sent by patients.

TTM allows the health care professional to assess transient conditions that cause such symptoms as palpitations, dizziness, syncope, confusion, paroxysmal dyspnea, and chest pain. Such conditions, which are commonly not apparent while the patient is with a health care professional, can make diagnosis difficult and costly.

With TTM, the patient can transmit an ECG recording from his home when the symptoms appear, avoiding the need to go to the health care facility and offering a better opportunity for early diagnosis. Even if symptoms seldom appear, the patient can keep the equipment for long periods, which further aids in the diagnosis of his condition.

Home care

TTM can also be used by a patient having cardiac rehabilitation at home. The patient is called regularly during this period to assess his progress. Because of this continuous monitoring, TTM can help reduce the anxiety felt by the patient and his family after discharge, especially if the patient suffered a myocardial infarction.

TTM is particularly valuable for assessing the effects of drugs and for diagnosing and managing paroxysmal arrhythmias. In both cases, TTM can eliminate the need for admitting the patient for evaluation and a potentially lengthy hospital stay.

TTM equipment

TTM requires three main pieces of equipment: an ECG recorder-transmitter, a standard telephone line, and a receiver. The ECG recorder-transmitter converts electrical activity from the patient's heart into acoustic waves. Some models contain built-in memory devices that store recordings of cardiac activity for transmission at a later time.

A standard telephone line is used to transmit information. The receiver converts the acoustic waves transmitted over the telephone line into ECG activity, which is then recorded on ECG paper for interpretation and documentation in the patient's chart. The recorder-transmitter uses two types of electrodes applied to the finger and chest. The electrodes produce ECG tracings similar to those of a standard 12-lead ECG.

Credit card–sized recorder

When a patient becomes symptomatic, he holds the back of the credit card-sized recorder (which operates on a battery) firmly to the center of his chest and pushes the START button. Four electrodes located on the back of the card sense electrical activity and record it. The card can store 30 seconds of activity and can later transmit the recording across telephone lines for evaluation by a health care professional.

■ *Limb leads*

The six limb leads record electrical activity in the heart's frontal plane, a view through the middle of the heart from top to bottom and right to left.

Viewing ECG leads

Each of the leads on a 12-lead electrocardiogram (ECG) views the heart from a different angle. These illustrations show the direction of electrical activity (depolarization) monitored by each lead and the corresponding 12 views of the heart.

Views reflected on a 12-lead ECG	Lead	View of the heart
	STANDARD LIMB LEADS (BIPOLAR)	
	I	Lateral wall
	II	Inferior wall
	III	Inferior wall
	AUGMENTED LIMB LEADS (UNIPOLAR)	
	aV_R	No specific view
	aV_L	Lateral wall
	aV_F	Inferior wall
	PRECORDIAL, OR CHEST, LEADS (UNIPOLAR)	
	V_1	Septal wall
	V_2	Septal wall
	V_3	Anterior wall
	V_4	Anterior wall
	V_5	Lateral wall
	V_6	Lateral wall

■ *Precordial leads*

The six precordial leads provide information on electrical activity in the heart's horizontal plane, a transverse view through the middle of the heart, dividing it into upper and lower portions.

■ *Electrical axes*

As well as assessing 12 different leads, a 12-lead ECG records the heart's electrical axis. The term *axis* refers to the direction of depolarization as it spreads through the heart. As impulses travel through the heart, they generate small electrical forces called *instantaneous vectors*. The mean of these vectors represents the force and direction of the wave of depolarization through the heart — the electrical axis. The electrical axis is also called the *mean instantaneous vector* and the *mean QRS vector*.

In a healthy heart, impulses originate in the sinoatrial node, travel through the atria to the atrioventricular node, and then travel to the ventricles. Most of the movement of the impulses is downward and to the left, the direction of a normal axis.

In an unhealthy heart, axis direction varies. That's because the direction of electrical activity travels away from areas of damage or necrosis and toward areas of hypertrophy. Knowing the normal deflection of each lead will help you evaluate whether the electrical axis is normal or abnormal.

■ *Obtaining a 12-lead ECG*

To perform a 12-lead ECG, you'll need to prepare properly, select the appropriate electrode sites, understand how to perform variations on a standard 12-lead ECG, and make an accurate recording.

PREPARATION

Gather all necessary supplies, including the ECG machine, recording paper, electrodes, and gauze pads. Tell the patient that the physician has ordered an ECG, and explain the procedure. Emphasize that the test takes about 10 minutes and that it's a safe and painless way to evaluate the heart's electrical activity. Answer the patient's questions, and offer reassurance. Preparing the patient properly will help alleviate anxiety and promote cooperation.

Ask the patient to lie in a supine position in the center of the bed with arms at his sides. If he can't tolerate lying flat, raise the head of the bed to the semi-Fowler's position. Document the patient's position during the procedure. Ensure privacy, and expose the patient's arms, legs, and chest, draping for comfort.

SITE SELECTION

Select the areas where you'll apply the electrodes. Choose areas that are flat and fleshy, not muscular or bony. Clip any excessive hair from the area. Remove excess oil and other substances such as body lotion from the skin to enhance electrode contact. Remember, the better the electrode contact is, the better the recording will be.

The 12-lead ECG provides 12 different views of the heart, just as 12 photographers snapping the same picture would produce 12 different photographs. Taking all of those snapshots requires placing four electrodes on the limbs and six across the front of the chest wall.

To help ensure an accurate recording, the electrodes must be applied correctly. Inaccurate placement of an electrode by greater than ⅝″ (1.5 cm) from its standardized position may lead to inaccurate waveforms and an incorrect ECG interpretation.

You'll need patience when obtaining a pediatric ECG. With the help of the parents, if possible, try distracting the attention of the child. If artifact from arm and leg movement is a problem, try placing the electrodes in a more proximal position on the extremity.

Limb lead placement

To record the bipolar limb leads I, II, and III and the unipolar limb leads aV_R, aV_L, and aV_F, place electrodes on both of the patient's arms and on his left leg. The right leg also receives an electrode, but that electrode acts as a ground and doesn't contribute to the waveform. (See *Limb lead placement.*)

Placing the electrodes on the patient is typically easy because each leadwire is labeled or color-coded. For example, a wire (usually white) might be labeled "RA" for right arm. Another (usually red) might be labeled "LL" for left leg.

Precordial lead placement

Precordial leads are also labeled or color-coded according to which wire corresponds to which lead. To record the six precordial leads (V_1 through V_6), position the electrodes on specific areas of the anterior chest wall. (See *Precordial lead placement,* page 105.) If they're placed too low, the ECG tracing will be inaccurate.

- Place lead V_1 over the fourth intercostal space at the right sternal border. To find the space, locate the sternal notch at the second rib and feel your way down the sternal border until you reach the fourth intercostal space.
- Place lead V_2 just opposite V_1, over the fourth intercostal space at the left sternal border.
- Place lead V_4 over the fifth intercostal space at the left midclavicular line. Placing lead V_4 before V_3 makes it easier to see where to place lead V_3.
- Place lead V_3 midway between V_2 and V_4.
- Place lead V_5 over the fifth intercostal space at the left anterior axillary line.
- Place lead V_6 over the fifth intercostal space at the left midaxillary line. If you've placed leads V_4 through V_6 correctly, they should line up horizontally.

Additional types of ECG leads

In addition to the standard 12-lead ECG, two other types of ECG leads may be used for diagnostic purposes: the posterior-lead ECG and the right chest-lead ECG. These ECG leads use chest and posterior leads to assess areas that standard 12-lead ECGs can't.

Posterior-lead ECG

Because of lung and muscle barriers, the usual chest leads can't "see" the heart's posterior surface to record myocardial damage there. So, some physicians add three posterior leads to the 12-lead ECG: leads V_7, V_8, and V_9. These leads are placed opposite anterior leads V_4, V_5, and V_6, on

Limb lead placement

Proper lead placement is critical for the accurate recording of cardiac rhythms. The diagrams here show electrode placement for the six limb leads. RA indicates right arm; LA, left arm; RL, right leg; and LL, left leg. The plus sign (+) indicates the positive pole, the minus sign (–) indicates the negative pole, and G indicates the ground. Below each diagram is a sample electrocardiogram recording for that lead.

LEAD I

Lead I connects the right arm (negative pole) with the left arm (positive pole).

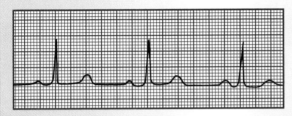

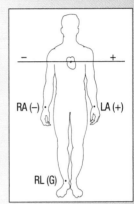

LEAD II

Lead II connects the right arm (negative pole) with the left leg (positive pole).

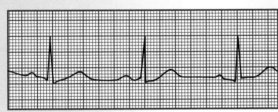

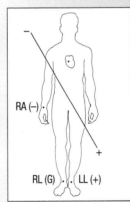

LEAD III

Lead III connects the left arm (negative pole) with the left leg (positive pole).

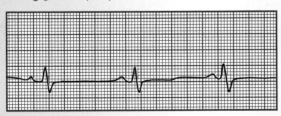

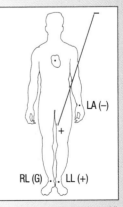

(continued)

Limb lead placement *(continued)*

LEAD aV$_R$
Lead aV$_R$ connects the right arm (positive pole) with the heart (negative pole).

LEAD aV$_L$
Lead aV$_L$ connects the left arm (positive pole) with the heart (negative pole).

LEAD aV$_F$
Lead aV$_F$ connects the left leg (positive pole) with the heart (negative pole).

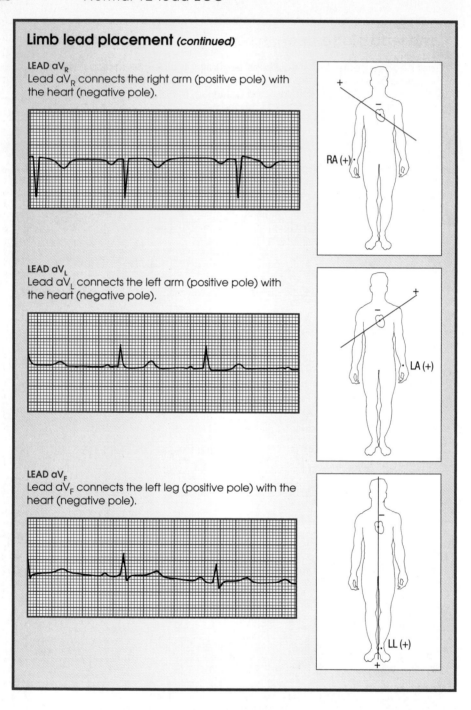

the left side of the patient's back, following the same horizontal line. (See *Posterior lead placement,* page 106.)

Occasionally, a physician may request right-sided posterior leads. These leads are labeled V$_{7R}$, V$_{8R}$, and V$_{9R}$ and are placed on the right

Precordial lead placement

The precordial leads complement the limb leads to provide a complete view of the heart. To record the precordial leads, place the electrodes as shown.

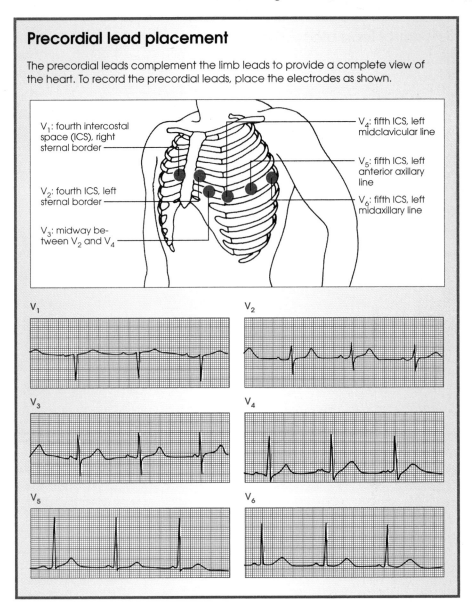

V_1: fourth intercostal space (ICS), right sternal border

V_2: fourth ICS, left sternal border

V_3: midway between V_2 and V_4

V_4: fifth ICS, left midclavicular line

V_5: fifth ICS, left anterior axillary line

V_6: fifth ICS, left midaxillary line

V_1

V_2

V_3

V_4

V_5

V_6

side of the patient's back. Their placement is a mirror image of the electrodes on the left side of the back. This type of ECG provides information on the right posterior area of the heart.

Right chest-lead ECG

The standard 12-lead ECG evaluates only the left ventricle. If the right ventricle needs to be assessed for damage or dysfunction, the physician may order a right chest-lead ECG. For example, a patient with an inferior wall MI might have a right chest-lead ECG to rule out right ventricular involvement.

Posterior lead placement

Posterior leads can be used to assess the heart's posterior surface. To ensure an accurate reading, make sure the posterior electrodes V_7, V_8, and V_9 are placed at the same horizontal level as the V_6 lead at the fifth intercostal space. Place lead V_7 at the posterior axillary line, lead V_9 at the paraspinal line, and lead V_8 halfway between leads V_7 and V_9.

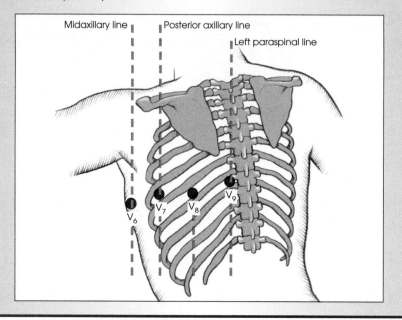

With this type of ECG, the six leads are placed on the right side of the chest in a mirror image of the standard precordial lead placement. Electrodes start at the left sternal border and swing down under the right breast area. (See *Right precordial lead placement.*)

RECORDING THE ECG

After properly placing the electrodes, record the ECG. ECG machines come in two types: multichannel recorders (most common) and single-channel recorders. With a multichannel recorder, all electrodes are attached to the patient at once and the machine prints a simultaneous view of all leads. With a single-channel recorder, one lead at a time is recorded in a short strip by attaching and removing electrodes and stopping and starting the tracing each time. (See *Normal findings in a 12-lead ECG,* pages 108 to 111.)

To record a multichannel ECG, follow these steps:

■ Plug the cord of the ECG machine into a grounded outlet. If the machine operates on a charged battery, it may not need to be plugged in.

■ Place all of the electrodes on the patient.

Right precordial lead placement

Right precordial leads can provide specific information about the function of the right ventricle. Place the six leads on the right side of the chest in a mirror image of the standard precordial lead placement, as shown here.

V_{1R}: fourth intercostal space (ICS), left sternal border
V_{2R}: fourth ICS, right sternal border
V_{3R}: halfway between V_{2R} and V_{4R}
V_{4R}: fifth ICS, right midclavicular line
V_{5R}: fifth ICS, right anterior axillary line
V_{6R}: fifth ICS, right midaxillary line

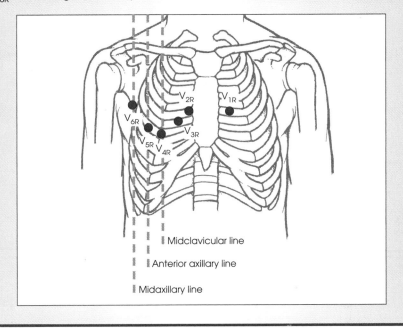

■ Make sure all leads are securely attached, and then turn on the machine.

■ Instruct the patient to relax, lie still, and breathe normally. Ask him not to talk during the recording, to prevent distortion of the ECG tracing.

■ Set the ECG paper speed selector to 25 mm per second. If necessary, enter the patient's identification data.

■ Press the appropriate button on the ECG machine and record the ECG.

■ Observe the quality of the tracing. When the machine finishes the recording, turn it off.

■ Remove the electrodes, and clean the patient's skin.

(Text continues on page 111.)

Normal findings in a 12-lead ECG

Each electrocardiogram (ECG) waveform (P wave, QRS complex, T wave) represents the electrical events occurring in one cardiac cycle. The 12-lead ECG provides 12 views of the electrical activity of the heart, which includes three bipolar leads (I, II, and III), three unipolar augmented leads (aV_R, aV_L, and aV_F), and six precordial, or chest, leads (V_1, V_2, V_3, V_4, V_5, and V_6). Each lead on a 12-lead ECG views the heart from a different angle. The tracings shown here represent normal findings of the heart's electrical activity in each of the 12 leads.

LEAD I

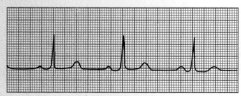

P wave: Upright
Q wave: Small or none
R wave: Largest wave
S wave: None present, or smaller than R wave
T wave: Upright
U wave: None present
ST segment: Usually isoelectric, but may vary from +1 to –0.5 mm

LEAD II

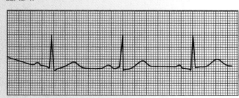

P wave: Upright
Q wave: Small or none
R wave: Large (vertical heart)
S wave: None present, or smaller than R wave
T wave: Upright
U wave: None present
ST segment: Usually isoelectric, but may vary from +1 to –0.5 mm

LEAD III

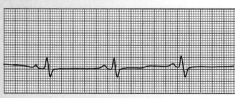

P wave: Upright, diphasic, or inverted
Q wave: Usually small or none (a Q wave must also be present in lead aV_F to be considered diagnostic)
R wave: None present to large wave
S wave: None present to large wave, indicating horizontal heart
T wave: Upright, diphasic, or inverted
U wave: None present
ST segment: Usually isoelectric, but may vary from +1 to –0.5 mm

Normal findings in a 12-lead ECG *(continued)*

LEAD aV$_R$

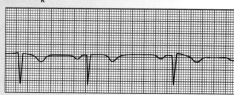

P wave: Inverted
Q wave: None, small wave, or large wave present
R wave: None, or small wave present
S wave: Large wave (may be QS)
T wave: Inverted
U wave: None present
ST segment: Usually isoelectric, but may vary from +1 to –0.5 mm

LEAD aV$_L$

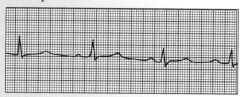

P wave: Upright, diphasic, or inverted
Q wave: None, small wave, or large wave present (a Q wave must also be present in lead I or precordial leads to be considered diagnostic)
R wave: None, small wave, or large wave present (large wave indicates horizontal heart)
S wave: None present to large wave (large wave indicates vertical heart)
T wave: Upright, diphasic, or inverted
U wave: None present
ST segment: Usually isoelectric, but may vary from +1 to –0.5 mm

LEAD aV$_F$

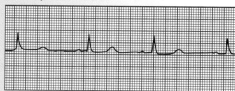

P wave: Upright
Q wave: None, or small wave present
R wave: None, small wave, or large wave present (large wave suggests vertical heart)
S wave: None present to large wave (large wave suggests horizontal heart)
T wave: Upright, diphasic, or inverted
U wave: None present
ST segment: Usually isoelectric, but may vary from +1 to –0.5 mm

(continued)

Normal findings in a 12-lead ECG *(continued)*

LEAD V₁

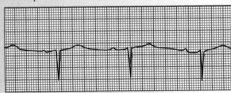

P wave: Upright, diphasic, or inverted
Q wave: Deep QS pattern possibly present
R wave: None present, or less than S wave
S wave: Large (part of QS pattern)
T wave: Usually inverted, but may be upright and diphasic
U wave: None present
ST segment: May vary from 0 to +1 mm

LEAD V₂

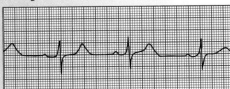

P wave: Upright
Q wave: Deep QS pattern possibly present
R wave: None present, or less than S wave (wave may become progressively larger)
S wave: Large (part of QS pattern)
T wave: Upright
U wave: Upright; lower amplitude than T wave
ST segment: May vary from 0 to +1 mm

LEAD V₃

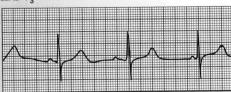

P wave: Upright
Q wave: None, or small wave present
R wave: Less than, greater than, or equal to S wave (wave may become progressively larger)
S wave: Large (greater than R wave, less than R wave, or equal to R wave)
T wave: Upright
U wave: Upright; lower amplitude than T wave
ST segment: May vary from 0 to +1 mm

Normal findings in a 12-lead ECG *(continued)*

LEAD V₄

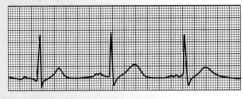

P wave: Upright
Q wave: None, or small wave present
R wave: Progressively larger wave; R wave greater than S wave
S wave: Progressively smaller (less than R wave)
T wave: Upright
U wave: Upright; lower amplitude than T wave
ST segment: Usually isoelectric, but may vary from +1 to –0.5 mm

LEAD V₅

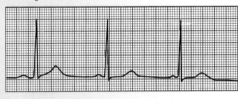

P wave: Upright
Q wave: Small
R wave: Progressively larger, but less than 26 mm
S wave: Progressively smaller; less than the S wave in V₄
T wave: Upright
U wave: None present
ST segment: Usually isoelectric, but may vary from +1 to –0.5 mm

LEAD V₆

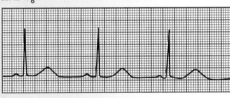

P wave: Upright
Q wave: Small
R wave: Largest wave, but less than 26 mm
S wave: Smallest wave; less than the S wave in V₅
T wave: Upright
U wave: None present
ST segment: Usually isoelectric, but may vary from +1 to –0.5 mm

ECG PRINTOUT

Depending on the information entered, ECG printouts from a multichannel ECG machine will show the patient's name, room number and, possibly, medical record number. At the top of the printout, you'll see the patient's heart rate and wave durations, measured in seconds. (See *Reading the multichannel ECG recording,* page 112.)

Some machines can record ST-segment elevation and depression. The name of the lead will appear next to each 6-second strip.

Reading the multichannel ECG recording

The top of a 12-lead electrocardiogram (ECG) recording usually shows patient identification information along with an interpretation by the machine. A rhythm strip is commonly included at the bottom of the recording.

Standardization

Look for standardization marks on the recording, normally 10 small squares high. If the patient has high voltage complexes, the marks will be half as high. You'll also notice that lead markers separate the lead recordings on the paper and that each lead is labeled.

Familiarize yourself with the order in which the leads are arranged on an ECG tracing. Getting accustomed to the layout of the tracing will help you interpret the ECG more quickly and accurately.

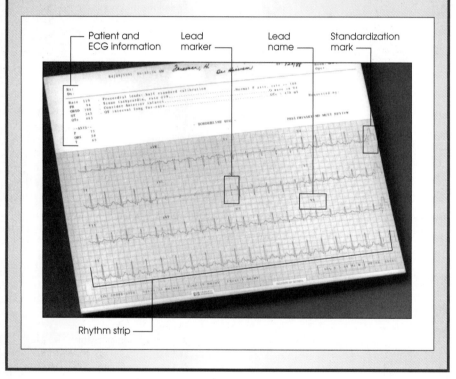

If not already included on the printout, be sure to write the following information: date, time, physician's name, and special circumstances. For example, you might record an episode of chest pain, abnormal electrolyte levels, related drug treatment, abnormal placement of the electrodes, or the presence of an artificial pacemaker and whether a magnet was used while the ECG was obtained.

Remember, ECGs are legal documents. They belong in the patient's medical record and must be saved for future reference and comparison with baseline strips.

6 *Electrical axis determination*

■ *Electrical axis*

The *electrical axis* is the average direction of the heart's electrical activity during ventricular depolarization. Leads placed on the body sense the sum of the heart's electrical activity and record it as waveforms.

You can determine your patient's electrical axis by examining the waveforms recorded from the six frontal plane leads: I, II, III, aV_R, aV_L, and aV_F. Imaginary lines drawn from each of the leads intersect at the center of the heart and form a diagram known as the *hexaxial reference system*. (See *Understanding the hexaxial reference system,* page 114.)

An axis that falls between 0 and 90 degrees is considered normal (some sources consider –30 to 90 degrees to be normal). An axis between 90 and 180 degrees indicates right axis deviation, and one between 0 and –90 degrees indicates left axis deviation (some sources consider –30 to –90 degrees to be left axis deviation). An axis between –180 and –90 degrees indicates extreme right axis deviation and is called an *indeterminate axis*.

In the neonate, right axis deviation, between +60 and +160 degrees, is normal due to dominance of the right ventricle. By age 1, the axis shifts to fall between +10 and +100 degrees as the left ventricle becomes dominant.

In elderly patients, left axis deviation commonly occurs. This axis shift may result from fibrosis of the anterior fascicle of the left bundle branch and because the thickness of the left ventricular wall increases by 25% between ages 30 and 80.

ELECTRICAL AXIS DETERMINATION
To determine your patient's electrical axis, use the *quadrant method* or the *degree method*.

Quadrant method
The quadrant method, a fast, easy way to plot the heart's axis, involves observing the main deflection of the QRS complex in leads I and aV_F. (See *Determining the quadrant method,* page 115.) Lead I indicates

113

Understanding the hexaxial reference system

The hexaxial reference system consists of six bisecting lines, each representing one of the six limb leads, and a circle, representing the heart. The intersection of all lines divides the circle into equal, 30-degree segments.

Shifting degrees

Note that 0 degrees appears at the 3 o'clock position (positive pole lead I). Moving counter-clockwise, the degrees become increasingly negative, until reaching ±180 degrees, at the 9 o'clock position (negative pole lead I).

The bottom half of the circle contains the corresponding positive degrees. However, a positive-degree designation doesn't necessarily mean that the pole is positive.

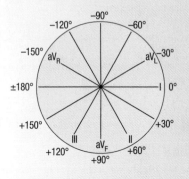

whether impulses are moving to the right or left, and lead aV_F indicates whether they're moving up or down.

If the QRS-complex deflection is positive or upright in both leads, the electrical axis is normal. If lead I is upright and lead aV_F points down, left axis deviation exists.

When lead I points down and lead aV_F is upright, right axis deviation exists. Both waves pointing down signal extreme right axis deviation.

Degree method

A more precise axis calculation, the degree method provides an exact measurement of the electrical axis. (See *Determining the degree method*, page 116.) It also allows you to determine the axis even if the QRS complex isn't clearly positive or negative in leads I and aV_F. To use this method, follow these four steps.

■ Review all six limb leads, and identify the one that contains either the smallest QRS complex or the complex with an equal deflection above and below the baseline.

■ Use the hexaxial diagram to identify the lead perpendicular to this lead. For example, if lead I has the smallest QRS complex, then the lead perpendicular to the line representing lead I would be lead aV_F.

■ After you've identified the perpendicular lead, examine its QRS complex. If the electrical activity is moving toward the positive pole of a lead, the QRS complex deflects upward. If it's moving away from the positive pole of a lead, the QRS complex deflects downward.

■ Plot this information on the hexaxial diagram to determine the direction of the electrical axis.

Determining the quadrant method

This chart will help you quickly determine the direction of a patient's electrical axis. Observe the deflections of the QRS complexes in leads I and aV$_F$. Then check the chart to determine whether the patient's axis is normal or has a left, right, or extreme right axis deviation.

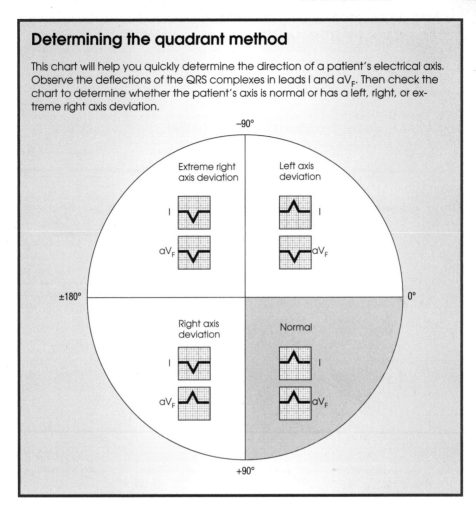

AXIS DEVIATION

Finding a patient's electrical axis can help confirm a diagnosis or narrow the range of possible diagnoses. Factors that influence the location of the axis include the heart's position in the chest, the heart's size, the patient's body size or type, the conduction pathways, and the force of the electrical impulses being generated. Causes of *left axis deviation* include:

- normal variation
- inferior wall myocardial infarction (MI)
- left anterior hemiblock
- Wolff-Parkinson-White syndrome
- mechanical shifts (ascites, pregnancy, tumors)
- left bundle-branch block
- left ventricular hypertrophy
- aortic stenosis
- aging.

Determining the degree method

The degree method of determining axis deviation allows you to identify a patient's electrical axis by degrees on the hexaxial system, not just by quadrant. To use this method, take the following steps.

Step 1
Identify the limb lead with the smallest QRS complex or the equiphasic QRS complex. In this example, it's lead III.

LEAD I	LEAD II	LEAD III

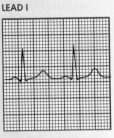 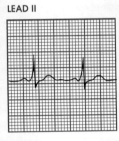 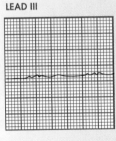

LEAD aV$_R$	LEAD aV$_L$	LEAD aV$_F$

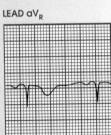 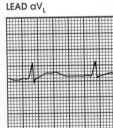 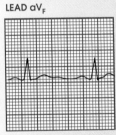

Step 2
Locate the axis for lead III on the hexaxial diagram. Then find the axis perpendicular to it, which is the axis for lead aV$_R$.

Step 3
Now, examine the QRS complex in lead aV$_R$, noting whether the deflection is positive or negative. As you can see, the QRS complex for this lead is negative, indicating that the current is moving toward the negative pole of aV$_R$, which is in the right lower quadrant at +30 degrees on the hexaxial diagram. So the electrical axis here is normal at +30 degrees.

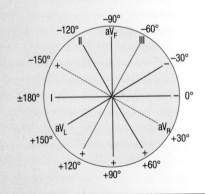 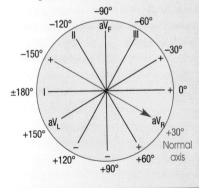

Causes of *right axis deviation* include:
- normal variation
- lateral wall MI
- left posterior hemiblock
- right bundle-branch block (RBBB)
- emphysema
- right ventricular hypertrophy
- pulmonary hypertension
- pulmonic stenosis.

Remember that electrical activity in the heart swings away from areas of damage or necrosis, so the damaged part of the heart will be the last area depolarized. For example, in RBBB, the impulse travels quickly down the normal left side and then moves slowly down the right side. This shifts the electrical forces to the right, causing right axis deviation.

Axis deviation isn't always clinically significant, and it isn't always cardiac in origin. For example, infants and children typically have right axis deviation. Pregnant women typically have left axis deviation.

7 *Acute coronary syndromes*

A 12-lead electrocardiogram (ECG) is used to assist in the diagnosis of certain conditions such as unstable angina, myocardial infarction, and pericarditis. By reviewing sample ECGs, you'll know the classic signs to look for. This chapter examines ECG characteristics of each of these cardiac conditions.

■ *Acute coronary syndromes*

Acute myocardial infarction (MI) (ST-segment elevation MI [STEMI] and non–ST-segment elevation MI [NSTEMI]) and unstable angina are now recognized as part of a group of clinical diseases called *acute coronary syndromes* (ACSs).

Rupture or erosion of plaque — an unstable and lipid-rich substance — initiates all coronary syndromes. The rupture results in platelet adhesions, fibrin clot formation, and activation of thrombin. (See *Understanding thrombus formation.*)

Early thrombus doesn't necessarily block coronary blood flow. When the thrombus does progress and occludes blood flow, an ACS results.

The degree of blockage and the time that the affected vessel remains occluded are major determinants for the type of infarct that occurs.

For patients with unstable angina, a thrombus partially occludes a coronary vessel. This thrombus is full of platelets. The partially occluded vessel may have distal microthrombi that cause necrosis in some myocytes. These patients may progress to a non–ST-segment elevation MI.

If a thrombus fully occludes the vessel for a prolonged time, this is known as an *ST-segment elevation MI*. In this type of MI, there's a greater concentration of thrombin and fibrin.

CAUSES OF ACS

Causes of ACS include atherosclerosis and embolus. In atherosclerosis, plaque forms and subsequently ruptures or erodes, resulting in platelet adhesions, fibrin clot formation, and activation of thrombin.

Risk factors for ACS include:
■ diabetes

Understanding thrombus formation

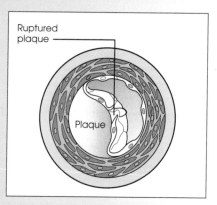

1. Plaque in coronary artery ruptures or erodes.

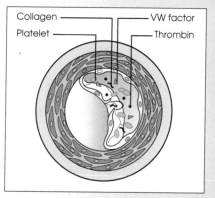

2. Platelets adhere to damaged area and become exposed to activating factors (collagen, thrombin, von Willebrand (VW) factor).

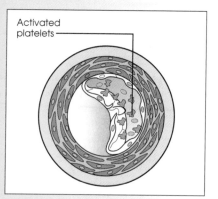

3. Platelet activation produces glycoprotein IIb and IIIa receptors that bind fibrinogen.

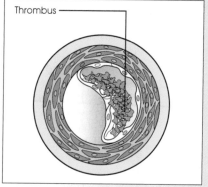

4. Platelet aggregation and adhesion continue, enlarging thrombus.

- family history of heart disease
- high-fat, high-carbohydrate diet
- hyperlipoproteinemia
- hypertension
- menopause
- obesity
- sedentary lifestyle
- smoking
- stress
- inflammation.

SIGNS AND SYMPTOMS
Angina
A patient with *angina* typically experiences burning, squeezing, and a crushing tightness in the substernal or precordial chest that may radiate to the left arm, neck, jaw, or shoulder blade.

Angina usually follows physical exertion, but may also follow emotional excitement, exposure to cold, or a large meal. Angina has four major forms, although only unstable angina is classified under acute coronary syndromes.

■ *Stable angina* — pain is predictable in frequency and duration, and it can be relieved with nitroglycerin and rest.

■ *Unstable angina* — pain increases in frequency and duration and is more easily induced, which indicates a worsening of coronary artery disease and may progress to MI.

■ *Prinzmetal's* (or *variant*) *angina* — pain is caused by unpredictable spasm of the coronary arteries; it may occur spontaneously and may not be related to physical exercise or emotional stress.

■ *Microvascular angina* — angina-like pain is due to impairment of vasodilator reserve in a patient with normal coronary arteries.

MI
Although other diagnoses may have chest pain as a symptom, retrosternal chest discomfort, pain, or pressure is a prime symptom of an infarction.

Patients typically describe these symptoms of acute ischemia and MI:

■ uncomfortable pressure, squeezing, burning, severe persistent pain, or fullness in the center of the chest lasting several minutes (usually longer than 15 minutes)

■ pain radiating to the shoulders, neck, arms, or jaws or pain in the back between the shoulder blades

■ accompanying symptoms of light-headedness, fainting, sweating, nausea, shortness of breath; anxiety, or a feeling of impending doom

■ most patients experience typical chest pain with acute ischemia and MI; but women, and occasionally men, elderly patients, and patients with diabetes may experience atypical chest pain. Atypical symptoms include upper back discomfort between the shoulder blades, palpitations, feeling of fullness in the neck, nausea, abdominal discomfort, dizziness, unexplained fatigue, and exhaustion or shortness of breath.

ECG CHARACTERISTICS
Angina
■ Most patients with angina show ischemic changes on an ECG only during the attack. (See *ECG changes associated with angina.*) Because these changes may be fleeting, always obtain an order for, and perform, a 12-lead ECG and, when necessary, additional posterior and right precordial ECG leads as soon as the patient reports chest pain.

■ The ECG will help you determine which area of the heart and which coronary arteries are involved. By recognizing danger early, you may be

ECG changes associated with angina

Illustrated below are some classic electrocardiogram (ECG) changes involving the T wave and ST segment that you may see when monitoring a patient with angina.

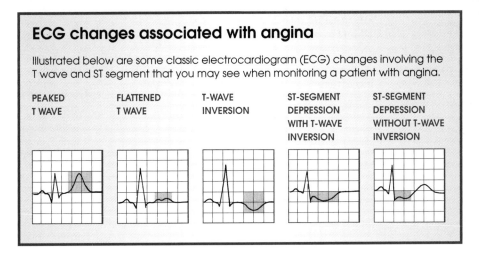

PEAKED T WAVE	FLATTENED T WAVE	T-WAVE INVERSION	ST-SEGMENT DEPRESSION WITH T-WAVE INVERSION	ST-SEGMENT DEPRESSION WITHOUT T-WAVE INVERSION

able to prevent MI or even death. (See *Recognizing Wellens syndrome,* pages 122 to 124.)

MI
■ The initial step in assessing a patient complaining of chest pain is to obtain an ECG. This should be done within 10 minutes of the patient's being seen by a health care professional. It's a crucial component in determining if myocardial ischemia is present. Interpretation of the ECG is the next step in identifying an ACS. The findings will direct the patient's treatment plan. (See *Stages of myocardial ischemia, injury, and infarct,* page 125).
■ According to the American Heart Association, patients should be classified as having ST-segment elevation or new left bundle-branch block (LBBB), ST-segment depression or dynamic T-wave inversion, or nondiagnostic or normal ECG.

ST-segment elevation or new LBBB
■ Patients with an ST-segment elevation greater than or equal to 1 mm in two or more leads or with new LBBB need to be treated for acute MI.
■ More than 90% of patients with this presentation will develop new Q waves and have positive serum cardiac markers.
■ Repeating the ECG may be helpful for patients who present with hyperacute T waves.
■ Patients with ST depression, which may indicate a posterior MI, benefit most when an acute MI diagnosis is confirmed. Posterior-lead ECG is used to confirm the diagnosis.

ST-segment depression or dynamic T-wave inversion
■ Ischemia should be suspected with findings of ST depression greater than or equal to 0.5 mm, marked symmetrical T-wave inversion in multiple precordial leads, and dynamic ST-T changes with pain.

Recognizing Wellens syndrome

Wellens syndrome occurs in about 14% to 18% of patients with unstable angina. Patients typically have a history of chest pain with normal or slightly elevated cardiac markers. The syndrome is characterized by specific ST-segment and T-wave changes that indicate a preinfarction state involving a critical proximal stenosis in the left anterior descending coronary artery. Identification and intervention of this syndrome before a myocardial infarction (MI) can reduce morbidity and mortality in these patients.

The characteristic precordial-lead electrocardiogram (ECG) changes include:
- no pathologic Q waves
- normal or minimally elevated ST segments
- T-wave changes:
The most common change (shown here) is a deep symmetrical T-wave inversion.

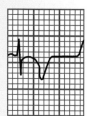 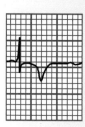

Less common is a biphasic T-wave pattern (shown here).

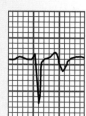 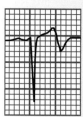

Typically, ECG changes in Wellens syndrome involve leads V_2 and V_3; however, occasionally all precordial leads V_1 through V_6 may be involved. These characteristic changes frequently occur when the patient isn't experiencing chest pain. Early identification of Wellens syndrome and treatment of coronary artery stenosis can prevent an acute MI.

Some patients experience a delay between the onset of pain and the appearance of certain ECG changes. Shown here are 12-lead ECGs for a patient with Wellens syndrome. The first tracing was recorded while the patient was experiencing chest pain. Yet, leads V_1, V_2, and V_3 show only slight T-wave changes (slight T-wave inversion at the end of the T wave). However, in the second tracing, which was taken 12 hours later when the patient was no longer experiencing pain, leads V_2 through V_6 show deeply inverted, symmetrical T waves and ST-segment abnormalities typical of Wellens syndrome.

Recognizing Wellens syndrome *(continued)*

ECG DURING ANGINAL PAIN

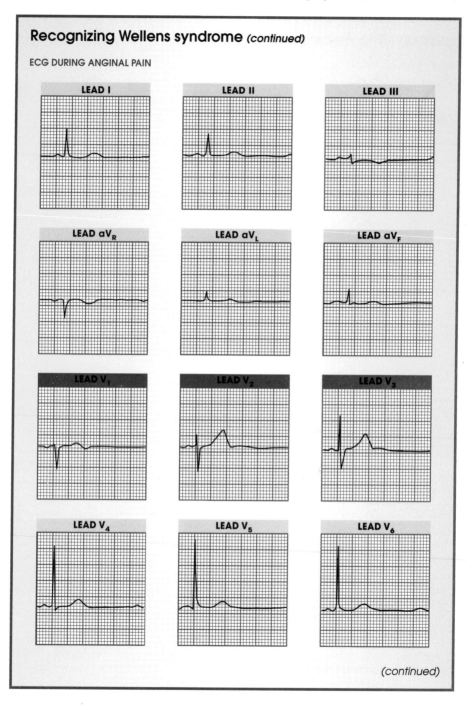

(continued)

■ Patients who display persistent symptoms and recurrent ischemia, diffuse or widespread ECG abnormalities, heart failure, and positive serum markers are considered high risk.

Recognizing Wellens syndrome *(continued)*

ECG AFTER CESSATION OF ANGINAL PAIN

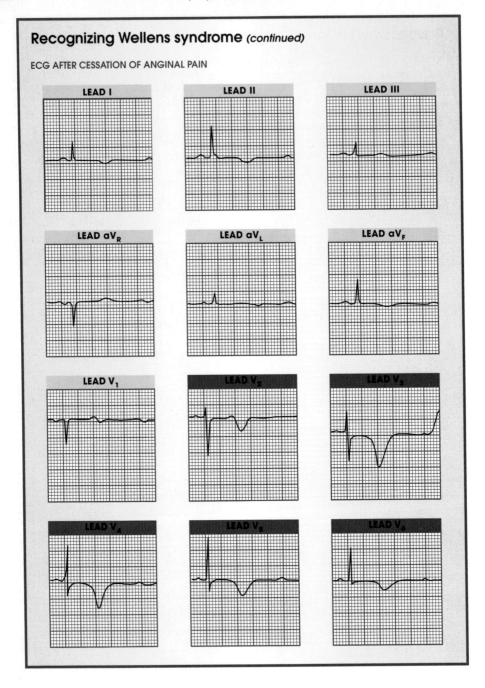

Nondiagnostic or normal ECG
- A normal ECG won't show any ST changes or arrhythmias.
- If the ECG is nondiagnostic, it may show an ST depression of less than 0.5 mm or a T-wave inversion or flattening in leads with dominant R waves.

Stages of myocardial ischemia, injury, and infarct

Three stages occur when there's occlusion of a vessel: ischemia, injury, and infarct:

Ischemia

Ischemia is the first stage and indicates that blood flow and oxygen demand are out of balance. It can be resolved by improving flow or reducing oxygen needs. Electrocardiogram (ECG) changes indicate ST-segment depression or T-wave changes.

Injury

The second stage, injury, occurs when the ischemia is prolonged enough to damage the area of the heart. ECG changes typically reveal ST-segment elevation (usually in two or more leads).

Infarct

Infarct is the third stage and occurs with actual death of myocardial cells. Scar tissue eventually replaces the dead tissue, and the damage caused is irreversible.

In the earliest stage of a myocardial infarction (MI), hyperacute or very tall and narrow T waves may be seen on the ECG. Within hours, the T waves become inverted and ST-segment elevation occurs in the leads facing the area of damage. The last change to occur in the evolution of an MI is the development of a pathologic Q wave, which is the only permanent ECG evidence of myocardial necrosis. Q waves are considered pathologic when they appear greater than or equal to 0.04 second wide and their height is greater than 25% of the R-wave height in that lead. Pathologic Q waves develop in over 90% of patients with ST-segment elevation MI. Approximately 25% of patients with non–ST-segment elevation MI will develop pathologic Q waves and the remaining patients will have a non–Q-wave MI.

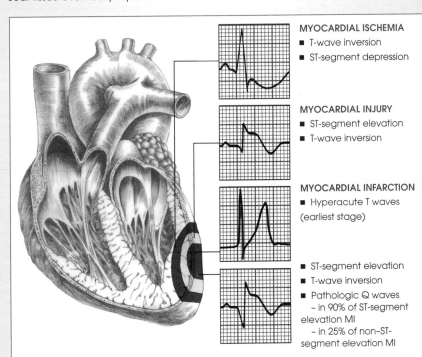

MYOCARDIAL ISCHEMIA
- T-wave inversion
- ST-segment depression

MYOCARDIAL INJURY
- ST-segment elevation
- T-wave inversion

MYOCARDIAL INFARCTION
- Hyperacute T waves (earliest stage)

- ST-segment elevation
- T-wave inversion
- Pathologic Q waves
  – in 90% of ST-segment elevation MI
  – in 25% of non–ST-segment elevation MI

Comparing MI with acute pericarditis

Myocardial infarction (MI) and acute pericarditis cause ST-segment elevation on an electrocardiogram (ECG). However, the ST segment and T wave (shaded areas) on an MI waveform are quite different from those on the pericarditis waveform.

In addition, because pericarditis involves the surrounding pericardium, several leads will show ST-segment and T-wave changes (typically leads I, II, aV_F, and V_4 through V_6). In MI, however, only those leads reflecting the area of infarction will show the characteristic changes.

These rhythm strips demonstrate the ECG variations between MI and acute pericarditis.

MI

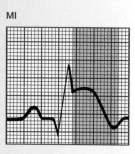

ACUTE PERICARDITIS

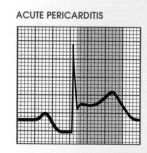

- Continue assessment of myocardial changes through use of serial ECGs, ST-segment monitoring, and serum cardiac markers.
- If further assessment is warranted, perform perfusion radionuclide imaging and stress echocardiography.
- The patient with acute pericarditis will also present with ST-segment elevation. Review the 12-lead ECG to help you determine if the patient is having an acute MI or has developed acute pericarditis. The patient with pericarditis will have ST-segment and T-wave changes in several leads; however, in acute MI the changes will be seen in the leads reflecting the area of infarction. (See *Comparing MI with acute pericarditis* and *Recognizing pericarditis*.)

INTERVENTIONS

Treatment goals for the patient experiencing an ACS include:
- reducing the amount of myocardial necrosis in those with ongoing infarction
- decreasing cardiac workload and increasing oxygen supply to the myocardium
- preventing major adverse cardiac events
- providing for rapid defibrillation when ventricular fibrillation or pulseless ventricular tachycardia is present.

Recognizing pericarditis

Pericarditis is an inflammation of the pericardium, the fibroserous sac that envelops the heart. Pericarditis can be either acute or chronic. The acute form may be fibrinous or effusive, with purulent, serous, or hemorrhagic exudate. Chronic constrictive pericarditis causes dense fibrous thickening of the pericardium. Possible causes of pericarditis include:

- viral, bacterial, or fungal disorders
- rheumatic fever
- autoimmune disorders
- complications of cardiac injury (myocardial infarction, cardiotomy).

Regardless of the form, pericarditis can cause cardiac tamponade if fluid accumulates too quickly. It can also cause heart failure if constriction occurs.

Electrocardiogram changes in acute pericarditis evolve through two stages:

- Stage 1 — Diffuse ST-segment elevations of 1 to 2 mm in most limb leads and most precordial leads reflect the inflammatory process. Upright T waves are present in most leads. The ST-segment and T-wave changes are typically seen in leads I, II, III, aV_L, aV_F, and V_2 through V_6.
- Stage 2 — As pericarditis resolves, the ST-segment elevation and accompanying T-wave inversion resolves in most leads.

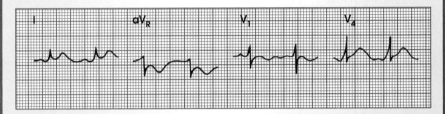

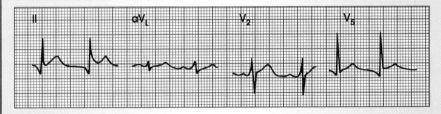

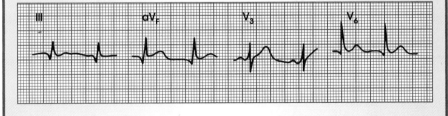

Release of cardiac enzymes and proteins

Because they're released by damaged tissue, serum proteins and isoenzymes (catalytic proteins that vary in concentration in specific organs) can help identify the compromised organ and assess the extent of damage. After acute myocardial infarction, cardiac enzymes and proteins rise and fall in a characteristic pattern, as shown in the graph below.

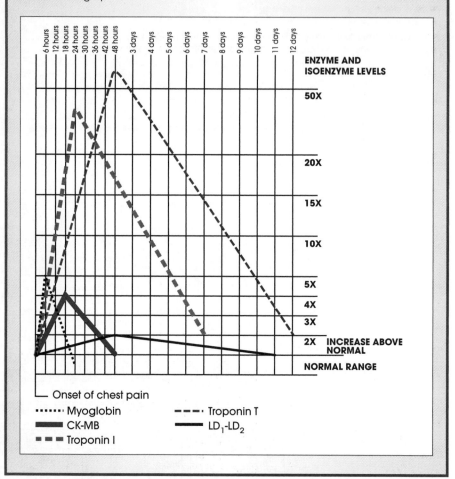

─ Onset of chest pain

⋯⋯ Myoglobin   ┈┈ Troponin T

━━ CK-MB   ━━ LD₁-LD₂

■■■ Troponin I

Initial treatment measures for ACS

Obtain a 12-lead ECG and additional posterior and right precordial leads as necessary, and serum cardiac markers as ordered to help confirm the diagnosis of acute MI. Serum cardiac markers (especially troponin I and CK-MB) are used to distinguish unstable angina and non–ST-segment elevation MI. (See *Release of cardiac enzymes and proteins*).

Use the mnemonic MONA, which stands for morphine, oxygen, nitroglycerin, and aspirin, to institute treatment for any patient experiencing ischemic chest pain or suspected ACS.

■ Give oxygen to increase oxygenation of blood.

- Give aspirin to inhibit platelet aggregation.
- Give nitroglycerin sublingually to relieve chest pain (unless systolic blood pressure is less than 90 mm Hg or heart rate is less than 50 beats/minute or greater than 100 beats/minute).
- Give morphine to relieve pain.

For the patient with unstable angina and non–ST-segment elevation MI, treatment includes the above initial measures as well as:
- beta-adrenergic blockers to reduce the heart's workload and oxygen demands
- heparin and glycoprotein IIb/IIIa inhibitors to minimize platelet aggregation and danger of coronary occlusion with high-risk patients (patients with planned cardiac catheterization and positive troponin)
- I.V. nitroglycerin to dilate coronary arteries and relieve chest pain (unless systolic blood pressure is less than 90 mm Hg or heart rate is less than 50 beats/minute or greater than 100 beats/minute)
- if the patient has an arrhythmia, prepare for use of antiarrhythmics, transcutaneous pacing patches (or transvenous pacemaker), or defibrillation
- percutaneous transluminal coronary angioplasty (PTCA) or coronary artery bypass graft (CABG) surgery for obstructive lesions
- antilipemic drugs to reduce elevated serum cholesterol or triglyceride levels.

For the patient with ST-segment elevation MI, treatment includes the above initial measures as well as:
- thrombolytic therapy (unless contraindicated) within 12 hours of onset of symptoms to restore vessel patency and minimize necrosis in ST-segment elevation MI
- I.V. heparin to promote patency in affected coronary artery
- beta-adrenergic blockers to reduce myocardial workload
- glycoprotein IIb/IIIa inhibitors to reduce platelet aggregation
- if the patient has an arrhythmia, prepare for use of antiarrhythmics, transcutaneous pacing patches (or transvenous pacemaker), or defibrillation
- angiotensin-converting enzyme inhibitors to reduce afterload and preload and prevent remodeling (begin in ST-segment elevation MI 6 hours after admission or when stable)
- interventional procedures, such as PTCA, stent placement, or surgical procedures, such as CABG, may open blocked or narrowed arteries.

■ *Types of myocardial infarction*

The location of the MI is a critical factor in determining the most appropriate treatment and predicting probable complications. Characteristic ECG changes that occur with each type of MI are localized to the leads overlying the infarction site. (See *Locating myocardial damage*, page 130.) This section takes a look at characteristic ECG changes that occur with different types of MIs.

Locating myocardial damage

After you've noted characteristic electrocardiogram lead changes in an acute myocardial infarction, use this table to identify the areas of damage. Match the lead changes (ST elevation, abnormal Q waves) in the second column with the affected wall in the first column and the artery involved in the third column. The fourth column shows reciprocal lead changes.

Wall affected	Leads	Artery involved	Reciprocal changes
Anterior	V_2, V_3, V_4	Left coronary artery, left anterior descending (LAD) artery	II, III, aV_F
Anterolateral	I, aV_L, V_2, V_3, V_4, V_5, V_6	LAD artery and diagonal branches, circumflex and marginal branches	II, III, aV_F
Anteroseptal	V_1, V_2, V_3, V_4	LAD artery	None
Inferior	II, III, aV_F	Right coronary artery (RCA)	I, aV_L
Lateral	I, aV_L, V_5, V_6	Circumflex branch of left coronary artery	II, III, aV_F
Posterior	V_8, V_9	RCA or circumflex	V_1, V_2, V_3, V_4 (R greater than S in V_1 and V_2, ST-segment depression, elevated T wave)
Right ventricular	V_{4R}, V_{5R}, V_{6R}	RCA	None

ANTERIOR WALL MI

The left anterior descending artery supplies blood to the anterior portion of the left ventricle, ventricular septum, and portions of the right and left bundle-branch systems.

When the left anterior descending artery becomes occluded, an anterior wall MI occurs. (See *Recognizing an anterior wall MI.*) Complications include second-degree atrioventricular blocks, bundle-branch blocks, ventricular irritability, and left-sided heart failure.

An anterior wall MI causes characteristic ECG changes in leads V_2 to V_4. The precordial leads show poor R-wave progression because the left ventricle can't depolarize normally. ST-segment elevation and T-wave inversion are also present.

The reciprocal leads for the anterior wall are the inferior leads II, III, and aV_F. They initially show tall R waves and depressed ST segments.

SEPTAL WALL MI

The patient with a septal wall MI is at increased risk for developing a ventricular septal defect. ECG changes are present in leads V_1 and V_2. In those leads, the R wave disappears, the ST segment rises, and the T wave

Recognizing an anterior wall MI

This 12-lead electrocardiogram shows typical characteristics of an anterior wall myocardial infarction (MI). Note that the R waves don't progress through the precordial leads. Also note the ST-segment elevation in leads V_2 and V_3. As expected, the reciprocal leads II, III, and aV_F show slight ST-segment depression. Axis is normal at +60 degrees.

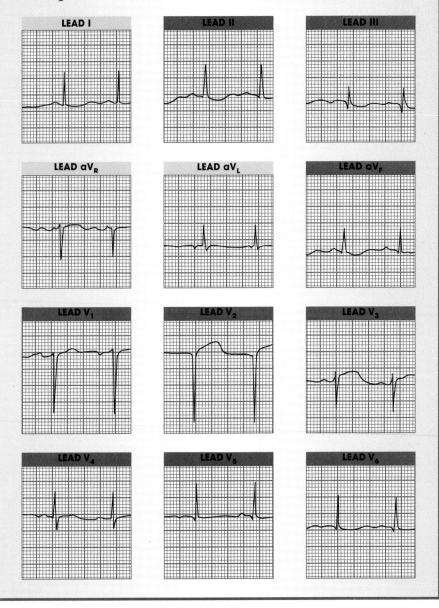

Recognizing a lateral wall MI

This 12-lead electrocardiogram shows typical characteristics of a lateral wall myocardial infarction (MI). Note the ST-segment elevation in leads I, aV_L, V_5, and V_6.

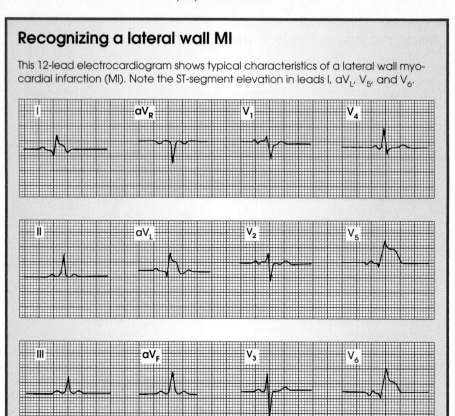

inverts. Because the left anterior descending artery also supplies blood to the ventricular septum, a septal wall MI typically accompanies an anterior wall MI.

LATERAL WALL MI

A lateral wall MI is usually caused by a blockage in the left circumflex artery and shows characteristic changes in the left lateral leads I, aV_L, V_5, and V_6. The reciprocal leads for a lateral wall infarction are leads II, III, and aV_F. (See *Recognizing a lateral wall MI*.)

A lateral wall MI typically causes premature ventricular contractions (PVCs) and varying degrees of heart block. It usually accompanies an anterior or inferior wall MI.

INFERIOR WALL MI

An inferior wall MI is usually caused by occlusion of the right coronary artery and produces characteristic ECG changes in the inferior leads II, III, and aV_F and reciprocal changes in the lateral leads I and aV_L. (See *Recognizing an inferior wall MI*.) It's also called a *diaphragmatic MI* because the inferior wall of the heart lies over the diaphragm.

Recognizing an inferior wall MI

This 12-lead electrocardiogram (ECG) shows the characteristic changes of an inferior wall myocardial infarction (MI). In leads II, III, and aV$_F$, note the T-wave inversion, ST-segment elevation, and pathologic Q waves. In leads I and aV$_L$, note the slight ST-segment depression — a reciprocal change. This ECG shows left axis deviation at –60 degrees.

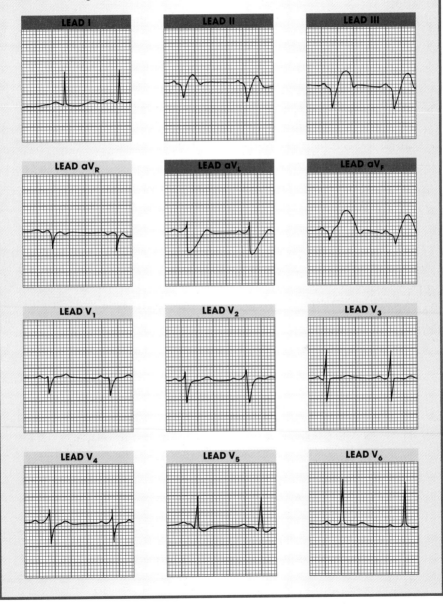

Recognizing a right ventricular MI

This 12-lead electrocardiogram shows typical characteristics of a right ventricular myocardial infarction (MI). Note the ST-segment elevation in the right precordial chest leads V_{4R}, V_{5R}, and V_{6R}. Pathologic Q waves would also appear in leads V_{4R}, V_{5R}, and V_{6R}.

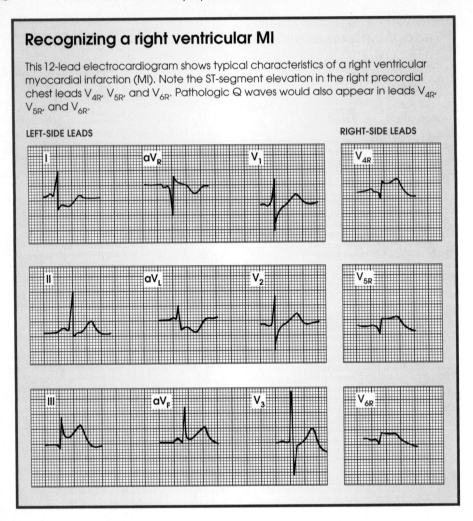

Patients with inferior wall MI are at risk for developing sinus bradycardia, sinus arrest, heart block, and PVCs. This type of MI occurs alone or with a lateral wall, posterior wall, or right ventricular MI.

POSTERIOR WALL MI

A posterior wall MI is caused by occlusion of the right coronary artery or the left circumflex arteries. It produces reciprocal changes in leads V_1 to V_4.

ECG changes for a posterior wall MI include tall R waves, ST-segment depression, and upright T waves. Posterior infarctions may accompany inferior infarctions. Data about the posterior wall and pathologic Q waves that might occur can be obtained from leads V_8 and V_9, using a posterior ECG.

RIGHT VENTRICULAR MI

A right ventricular MI usually follows occlusion of the right coronary artery. This type of MI rarely occurs alone. In 40% of patients, a right ventricular MI accompanies an inferior wall MI. (See *Recognizing a right ventricular MI.*)

A right ventricular MI can lead to right ventricular failure. The classic changes are ST-segment elevation, pathologic Q waves, and inverted T waves in the right precordial leads V_{2R} to V_{6R}. Identifying a right ventricular MI is difficult without information from the right precordial leads. If these leads aren't available, you can observe leads II, III, and aV_F or watch leads V_1 and V_2 for ST-segment elevation.

8 Bundle-branch block, enlargement, and hypertrophy

■ Bundle-branch block

With *bundle-branch block* (BBB), either the left or right bundle branch fails to conduct impulses normally. A BBB that occurs toward the distal end of the left bundle, in the posterior or anterior fasciculus, is called a *fascicular block* or *hemiblock*. Some blocks require treatment with a temporary pacemaker. Others are monitored only to detect whether they progress to a more complex block.

In BBB, the impulse travels down the unaffected bundle branch and then from one myocardial cell to the next to depolarize the ventricle. Because this cell-to-cell conduction progresses much more slowly than it does along the specialized cells of the conduction system, ventricular depolarization is prolonged.

Prolonged ventricular depolarization means that the QRS complex widens. The normal QRS duration is 0.06 to 0.10 second. A QRS complex duration more than 0.12 second may indicate that a BBB is present.

After identifying BBB, examine lead V_1 and lead V_6 on the 12-lead electrocardiogram (ECG). You'll use these leads to determine whether the block is in the right or left bundle branch.

Both temporary and permanent heart blocks may be associated with acute myocardial infarction (MI). An acute MI, in fact, is the primary cause of heart blocks. Other causes include atherosclerosis, valvular disease, ventricular hypertrophy, infective cardiac disease, congenital abnormalities, and cardiac drugs that alter the refractory period of interventricular conduction.

■ *Types of bundle-branch block*

The different types of heart blocks stem from different causes and have different implications for the patient. The different types include:
- right bundle-branch block (RBBB)
- left bundle-branch block (LBBB)
- left anterior fascicular block (LAFB) (also called *anterior hemiblock*)
- left posterior fascicular block (LPFB) (also called *posterior hemiblock*)
- trifascicular block.

With BBB, you may see an extra notch in the R wave, called *R prime (R'),* or an extra notch in the S wave, called *S prime (S').* And, of course, each type of BBB produces distinctive changes on a 12-lead ECG. Alternatively, you may see a QRS complex widened by a delta wave, a sign of preexcitation of the ventricle that occurs in Wolff-Parkinson-White syndrome. (See *Distinguishing WPW syndrome from BBB*, page 138.)

RIGHT BUNDLE-BRANCH BLOCK

When RBBB occurs, the impulse still activates the interventricular septum from left to right, but then the impulse activates the left ventricle before activating the right ventricle. (See *Understanding RBBB*, page 139.)

Causes

RBBB occurs with such conditions as anterior wall MI, coronary artery disease (CAD), and pulmonary embolism. Other causes include acute heart failure, rheumatic heart disease, valvular heart disease, right ventricular hypertrophy, hypokalemia, atrial septal defect, congenital anomalies, and cardiac catheterization of the right heart. It may also occur without cardiac disease. If it develops as the heart rate increases, it's called *rate-related RBBB*.

ECG characteristics

Rhythm: Atrial and ventricular rhythms regular
Rate: Atrial and ventricular rates within normal limits
P wave: May be normal in size and configuration
PR interval: Within normal limits
QRS complex: Duration appearing at least 0.12 second in complete block and 0.10 and 0.12 second in incomplete block. (In lead V_1, the QRS complex is wide and can appear in one of several patterns: an rSR′ complex with a wide S and R′ wave; an rSR′ complex with a wide R wave; and a wide R wave with an M-shaped pattern. The complex is mainly positive, with the R wave occurring late. In leads I, aV_L, and V_6, a broad S wave can be seen greater than 0.12 second and has a different configuration, sometimes resembling rabbit ears or the letter "M.") (See *Recognizing RBBB*, page 140.)
T wave: In most leads, deflection appearing opposite that of the QRS deflection

LOOK-ALIKES

Distinguishing WPW syndrome from BBB

Wolff-Parkinson-White (WPW) syndrome is a common type of preexcitation syndrome, an abnormal condition in which electrical impulses enter the ventricles from the atria by using an accessory pathway that bypasses the atrioventricular (AV) junction. This results in a short PR interval and a wide QRS complex with an initial slurring of the QRS complex, called a *delta wave*. Because the delta wave prolongs the QRS complex, its presence may be confused with a bundle-branch block (BBB).

WPW syndrome
■ A delta wave occurs at the beginning of the QRS complex, usually causing a distinctive slurring or hump in its initial slope. A delta wave isn't present in BBB.
■ On the 12-lead electrocardiogram (ECG), the delta wave will be most pronounced in the leads "looking at" the part of the heart where the accessory pathway is located.
■ The delta wave shortens the PR interval in WPW syndrome.

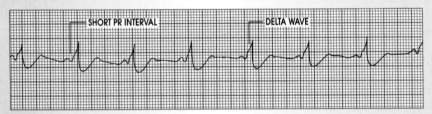

BBB
■ Carefully examine the QRS complex, noting which part of the complex is widened. A BBB involves a defective conduction of electrical impulses through the right or left bundle branch from the bundle of His to the Purkinje network, causing a right or left BBB.
■ This conduction disturbance results in an overall increase in QRS duration, or widening of the last part of the QRS complex, while the initial part of the QRS complex commonly appears normal.
■ Carefully examine the 12-lead ECG. With BBB, the prolonged duration of the QRS complexes will generally be consistent in all leads.
■ Measure the PR interval. BBB has no effect on the PR interval, so the PR intervals are generally normal. Keep in mind, though, that if the patient has a preexisting AV conduction defect, such as first-degree AV block, the PR interval will be prolonged.

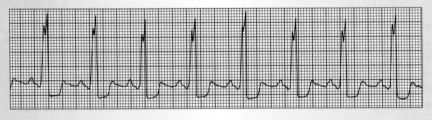

Understanding RBBB

In right bundle-branch block (RBBB), the initial impulse activates the interventricular septum from left to right, just as in normal activation (arrow 1). Next, the left bundle branch activates the left ventricle (arrow 2). The impulse then crosses the interventricular septum to activate the right ventricle (arrow 3).

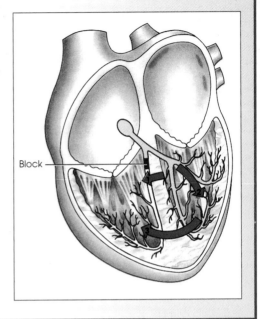

Block

QT interval: May be prolonged or within normal limits
Other: In precordial leads, triphasic complexes occurring because the right ventricle continues to depolarize after the left ventricle depolarizes, thereby producing a third phase of ventricular stimulation

Signs and symptoms

Typically there are no signs or symptoms of RBBB. Auscultation may reveal a fixed splitting of second heart sound (S$_2$).

Interventions

Treatment aims to correct the underlying problem. A pacemaker may be needed if RBBB occurs with an acute anteroseptal MI, especially if there's a preexisting left anterior or posterior fascicular block.

LEFT BUNDLE-BRANCH BLOCK

In LBBB, conduction through the left ventricle is impaired. A block may be located on the main bundle, or blocks may be located on both the anterior and posterior fascicles.

With LBBB, ventricular activation occurs in this order: First, the right ventricle is activated by the right bundle branch. Then the interventricular septum is activated abnormally in a right-to-left direction. And, finally, the left ventricle is activated. (See *Understanding LBBB*, page 141.)

Recognizing RBBB

This 12-lead electrocardiogram shows the characteristic changes of right bundle-branch block (RBBB). In lead V_1, note the rsR' pattern and T-wave inversion. In lead V_6, see the widened S wave and the upright T wave. Also note the prolonged QRS complexes.

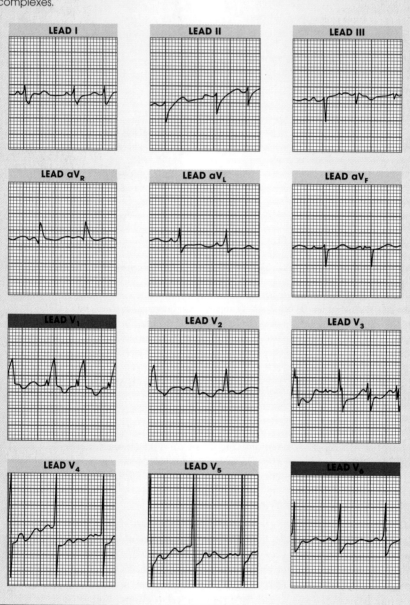

Understanding LBBB

In left bundle-branch block (LBBB), the impulse first travels down the right bundle branch (arrow 1). Then the impulse activates the interventricular septum from right to left (arrow 2), the opposite of normal activation. Finally, the impulse activates the left ventricle (arrow 3).

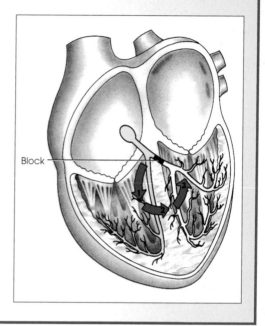

Block

Causes
When LBBB is discovered on a routine ECG, the patient may have hypertensive ischemic disease, primary heart disease, or no serious heart disease at all.

Severe CAD, hypertensive cardiovascular disease, and valvular disease represent the most common causes of LBBB. Cardiomyopathy, Lev's disease, Lenègre's disease, rheumatic disease, and congenital lesions may also produce LBBB.

ECG characteristics
Rhythm: Atrial and ventricular rhythms regular, depending on the underlying rhythm
Rate: Atrial and ventricular rates usually within normal limits
P wave: Normal in size and configuration
PR interval: Within normal limits
QRS complex: Duration varying from 0.10 and 0.12 second in incomplete LBBB; appearing at least 0.12 second in complete block; lead V_1 showing a wide, largely negative rS complex or entirely negative QS complex; leads I, AV_L, and V_6 showing a wide, tall R wave without a Q or S wave (See *Recognizing LBBB*, page 142.)
T wave: In most leads, deflection appearing opposite that of the QRS deflection
QT interval: May be prolonged or within normal limits

Recognizing LBBB

This 12-lead electrocardiogram shows characteristic changes of a left bundle-branch block (LBBB). All leads have prolonged QRS complexes. In lead V_1, note the QS wave pattern. In lead V_6, you'll see the wide and tall R wave and T-wave inversion. The elevated ST segments and upright T waves in leads V_1 to V_4 are also common in LBBB.

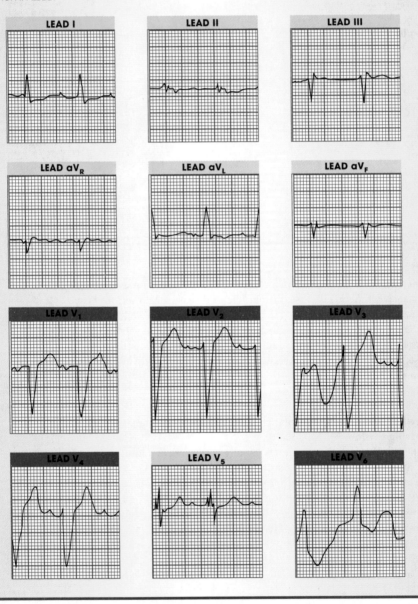

Understanding LAFB

In left anterior fascicular block (LAFB), the left ventricle is activated by the left posterior fascicle only (arrow 1), causing the impulse to be aimed downward and to the right initially. The right ventricle is depolarized by the right bundle branch at the same time (arrow 2). After the impulse reaches the Purkinje network, the impulse activates the anterior, lateral, and upper left ventricular walls (arrow 3).

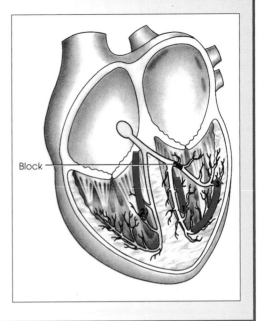

Block

Other: Magnitude of changes paralleling the magnitude of the QRS complex aberration; axis may be normal or showing left axis deviation; delayed intrinsicoid deflection over the left ventricle (lead V_6)

Signs and symptoms
Typically there are no signs or symptoms of LBBB. Auscultation may reveal a fixed splitting of S_2.

Interventions
Treatment aims to correct the underlying problem. For the patient who's had an acute MI, a pacemaker may be inserted because of the increased risk of complete atrioventricular (AV) block. A ventricular pacemaker may improve symptoms of heart failure in the patient with a large LBBB.

LEFT ANTERIOR FASCICULAR BLOCK
A blockage of the left anterior fascicle causes the left ventricle to be activated by the left posterior fascicle only. Impulses from this fascicle depolarize the inferior and posterior walls of the left ventricle. The right ventricle is depolarized by the right bundle branch at the same time. This depolarization causes the impulse to be aimed downward and to the right at first. After reaching the Purkinje network, the impulse activates the anterior, lateral, and upper left ventricular walls. (See *Understanding LAFB*.)

Recognizing LAFB

This 12-lead electrocardiogram shows characteristic changes of left anterior fascicular block (LAFB). Occurring in the anterosuperior fascicle of the left bundle branch, LAFB causes ventricular activation through the posteroinferior fascicle. As a result, left axis deviation takes place. Although less serious than a left posterior fascicular block, LAFB frequently occurs with right bundle-branch block or anterior myocardial infarction.

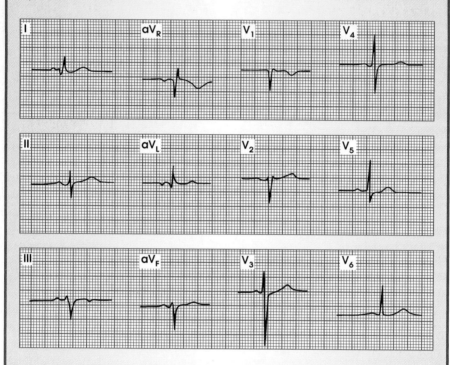

Causes

LAFB (also called *left anterior hemiblock*) can occur with an inferior wall MI, but it's more common with an acute anterior wall MI. LAFB can also result from CAD, hypertension, cardiomyopathies, and aortic valve disease. It's also associated with hyperkalemia, myocarditis, and degenerative conduction disorders, such as Lev's disease and Lenègre's disease. LAFB may also occur normally with aging.

ECG characteristics

Rhythm: Atrial and ventricular rhythms regular, depending on the underlying rhythm
Rate: Atrial and ventricular rates usually within normal limits
P wave: Normal in size and configuration
PR interval: Within normal limits
QRS complex: Duration appearing prolonged, but may fall within normal limits — 0.10 second or less; small Q wave appearing in lead I and

Understanding LPFB

In left posterior fascicular block (LPFB), the left anterior fascicle depolarizes the anterolateral wall of the left ventricle (arrow 1); at the same time, the right ventricle will be depolarized by the right bundle branch (arrow 2). After the impulse reaches the Purkinje network, it activates the inferoposterior wall of the left ventricle (arrow 3).

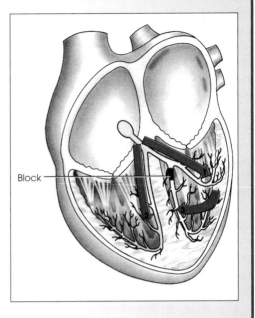

Block

a small R wave in lead III; a deep S wave in lead II; a deeper S wave in lead III; and an rS pattern in leads II and III (**See** *Recognizing LAFB.*)
QT interval: May be prolonged or within normal limits
T wave: May be inverted in leads I and aV_L and upright in leads II, III, and aV_F
Other: Left axis deviation usually –45 degrees or greater

Signs and symptoms
There are usually no signs and symptoms associated with LAFB.

Interventions
No treatment is usually necessary for LAFB. If the fascicular block occurs with an acute anteroseptal MI, a pacemaker may be required, especially if the patient has RBBB. If the patient has had an MI, monitor the modified chest lead (MCL_1) or V_1, and also watch for the development of RBBB.

LEFT POSTERIOR FASCICULAR BLOCK
With LPFB, the left anterior fascicle depolarizes the anterior and lateral walls of the left ventricle first. The right ventricle is depolarized by the right bundle branch at the same time. The impulse then crosses the Purkinje network and activates the inferior and posterior walls of the left ventricle. The impulse first moves to the left and anteriorly, then to the right and inferiorly. (See *Understanding LPFB.*)

Recognizing LPFB

This 12-lead electrocardiogram shows characteristic changes of left posterior fascicular block (LPFB). Occurring in the posteroinferior fascicle of the left bundle branch, LPFB causes ventricular activation through the anterosuperior fascicle. As a result, right axis deviation takes place. This arrhythmia is more serious than a left anterior fascicular block because it involves a larger lesion blocking the broad posterior fascicle. When a right bundle-branch block occurs with LPFB, it increases the likelihood of complete heart block.

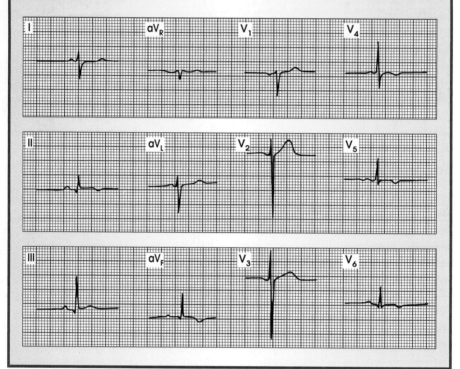

Causes

LPFB (also called *left posterior hemiblock*) usually occurs with an acute MI, ischemia, or CAD. Other causes include hypertension, aging, conduction system sclerosis, cardiomyopathy, and hyperkalemia.

ECG characteristics

Rhythm: Atrial and ventricular rhythms regular, depending on the underlying rhythm

Rate: Atrial and ventricular rates usually within normal limits

P wave: Normal in size and configuration

PR interval: Within normal limits

QRS complex: Duration appearing prolonged, but may fall within normal limits — 0.10 second or less; small Q wave appearing in leads III, a small R wave in lead I, and a deep S wave in lead I; large QRS complex in the precordial leads resulting from increased voltage (See *Recognizing LPFB*.)

T wave: May be inverted in leads I and aV_L and upright in leads II, III, and aV_F

QT interval: May be prolonged or within normal limits

Other: Mean QRS axis usually at least +120 degrees (right axis deviation) reflected by a negative lead I and a positive lead II

Signs and symptoms

There are usually no signs and symptoms associated with LPFB.

Interventions

No treatment is usually necessary for LPFB. If the fascicular block occurs with an acute anteroseptal MI, a pacemaker may be required, especially if the patient has RBBB. If the patient has had an MI, monitor MCL_1 or V_1, and watch for the development of RBBB also. If complete heart block results from RBBB with LPFB, treatment attempts to support and maintain a stable ventricular rhythm.

TRIFASCICULAR BLOCK

In trifascicular block, the intraventricular conduction abnormality involves the right bundle branch and also the anterior and posterior fascicles of the left bundle branch — it may be a form of complete heart block.

Causes

Trifascicular block may be caused by an MI, cardiac disease, or medications.

ECG characteristics

Trifascicular block exists when first-degree AV block is present in combination with LBBB involving both fascicles of the left bundle. Trifascicular block is also present when a first-degree AV block, along with RBBB and LAFB or LPFB, exists.

Signs and symptoms

Depending on the heart rate, the patient may experience syncope, dizziness, chest pain, or shortness of breath, or there may not be any signs or symptoms present.

Interventions

Treatment aims to correct the underlying condition. Usually, you'll also monitor the block in case it becomes more extensive. It's recommended to have a transcutaneous pacemaker on standby in the event that the patient develops complete heart block.

When RBBB occurs after an anterior wall MI, some physicians insert a temporary transvenous pacemaker as a prophylactic measure. A permanent pacemaker may be inserted if the condition is chronic.

■ *Enlargement and hypertrophy*

The atria and ventricles can enlarge because of an increase in pressure or increase in volume. The atria, which are thin-walled, usually dilate in response to an increase in pressure and an increase in volume. The ventricles, which are thick-walled, dilate with increased volume and hypertrophy with increased pressure.

Hypertrophy is an increase in the size of a cell or organ due to an increase in workload. Hypertrophy that occurs in the heart is thickening of the heart muscle as the muscle pumps against increasing resistance in the heart vessels, such as occurs with hypertension. This section discusses right and left atrial enlargement and right and left ventricular hypertrophy.

RIGHT ATRIAL ENLARGEMENT

Right atrial enlargement affects the P wave due to the initial part of the P wave occurring from right atrial depolarization.

Causes

Right atrial enlargement may be caused by chronic obstructive lung disease, tricuspid stenosis, tricuspid regurgitation, or pulmonary emboli.

ECG characteristics

Rhythm: Atrial and ventricular rhythms normal
Rate: Atrial and ventricular rates normal
P wave: Peaked P wave in lead II greater than 2.5 mm amplitude; V_1 increasing in initial positive deflection (See *Recognizing right atrial enlargement.*)
PR interval: Normal
QRS complex: QRS voltage in V_1 appearing less than 5 mm
ST segment: Normal
T wave: Normal
QT interval: Usually normal
Other: None

Signs and symptoms

Signs and symptoms are related to the underlying disorder.

Interventions

Treatment focuses on management of the underlying disorder such as hypertension.

Recognizing right atrial enlargement

The waveforms here show key electrocardiogram changes occurring in selected leads with right atrial enlargement.

In lead II, the P wave is tall and peaked (see highlighted area). In lead V_1, you'll see a biphasic P wave with an increase in the initial positive deflection followed by a smaller negative deflection (see highlighted area). In both leads, the P wave duration is increased.

LEAD II

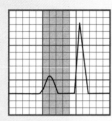

LEAD V_1

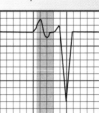

LEFT ATRIAL ENLARGEMENT

Left atrial enlargement causes delay in the electrical activity of the left atrium, resulting in a change in the shape of the P wave.

Causes

Left atrial enlargement may occur with mitral valve stenosis or mitral insufficiency. It also commonly occurs with any cause of left ventricular enlargement.

ECG characteristics

Rhythm: Atrial and ventricular rhythms normal
Rate: Atrial and ventricular rates normal
P wave: P wave duration of 0.11 msec or longer; notching of the P wave with the peaks being more than 1 mm apart and prominence of the terminal portion of the P wave, or prominent negativity of the terminal portion of the P wave in lead V_1 occurring (See *Recognizing left atrial enlargement,* page 150.)
PR interval: Normal
QRS complex: Normal
ST segment: Normal
T wave: Normal
QT interval: Usually normal

Recognizing left atrial enlargement

The waveforms here show key electrocardiogram changes occurring in selected leads with left atrial enlargement.

In lead II, the P wave is notched (see highlighted area). In lead V_1, you'll see a biphasic P wave with an initial positive deflection followed by a prominent negative deflection in the terminal portion of the wave (see highlighted area). In both leads, the P wave duration is increased.

LEAD II

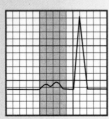

LEAD V_1

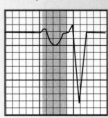

Signs and symptoms
Signs and symptoms are related to the underlying disorder.

Interventions
Treatment focuses on management of the underlying disorder such as hypertension.

RIGHT VENTRICULAR HYPERTROPHY
In *right ventricular hypertrophy* (RVH), the right ventricular wall thickens. RVH usually results from conditions that cause chronic increases in pressures within the ventricle.

Causes
RVH may occur as a result of right ventricle outflow obstruction, which may occur with pulmonary disease, primary pulmonary hypertension, pulmonary valve stenosis, tetralogy of Fallot, and ventricular septal defect.

ECG characteristics
Rhythm: Atrial and ventricular rhythms normal
Rate: Atrial and ventricular rates normal
P wave: May be normal in size and configuration, or may reflect right atrial enlargement
PR interval: Normal
QRS complex: R wave getting progressively smaller from V_1 to V_6 (normally it would increase) and there's a deep S wave in V_5 or V_6; normal or slightly increased QRS duration (See *Recognizing RVH.*)
ST segment: Depression may occur

Monophasic and biphasic defibrillators

There are two types of defibrillators: monophasic and biphasic.

Monophasic defibrillators

Monophasic defibrillators deliver a single current of electricity that travels in one direction between the two pads or paddles on the patient's chest. To be effective, a large amount of electrical current is required for monophasic defibrillation.

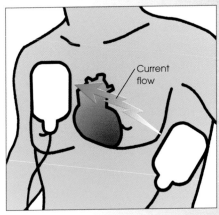

Current flow

Biphasic defibrillators

Biphasic defibrillators have pad or paddle placement, which is the same as the monophasic defibrillator. The difference is that during biphasic defibrillation, the electrical current discharged from the pads or paddles travels in a positive direction for a specified duration and then reverses and flows in a negative direction for the remaining time of the electrical discharge.

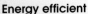

Current flow

Current flow

Energy efficient

The biphasic defibrillator delivers two currents of electricity and lowers the defibrillation threshold of the heart muscle, making it possible to successfully defibrillate ventricular fibrillation (VF) with smaller amounts of energy.

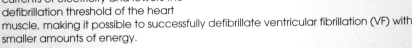
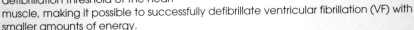

Adjustable

The biphasic defibrillator can adjust for differences in impedance or resistance of the current through the chest. This reduces the number of shocks needed to terminate VF.

Less myocardial damage

Because the biphasic defibrillator requires lower energy levels and fewer shocks, damage to the myocardial muscle is reduced. Biphasic defibrillators used at the clinically appropriate energy level may be used for defibrillation and, in the synchronized mode, for synchronized cardioversion.

Implantable cardioverter-defibrillator

An implantable cardioverter-defibrillator (ICD) continually monitors the heart for dangerous arrhythmias and administers shocks or paced beats to treat it.

Early ICDs (first used in 1980) could only deliver a shock to terminate VT and VF. However, today's advanced devices can detect a wide range of arrhythmias, including atrial fibrillation, bradycardia, ventricular tachycardia (VT), and ventricular fibrillation (VF).and automatically respond with the appropriate therapy, such as with bradycardia pacing (both single- and dual-chamber), antitachycardia pacing, cardioversion, or defibrillation shocks.

Nursing care
- Monitor the patient to ensure that the device is functioning properly.
- Provide emergency care, if indicated.
- Caution the patient to avoid large magnets, arc welders, large generators, and magnetic resonance imaging.
- Remind the patient about activity restrictions, if appropriate, such as swimming alone and driving.
- Recognize and promptly respond to complications after insertion, such as bleeding, pneumothorax, arrhythmias, and lead fracture.

Monitoring tips
When caring for a patient with an ICD, you should know how the device is programmed. This information is available on a status report. The report includes:
- type and model of ICD
- status of the device (on or off)
- detection rates
- therapies that will be delivered.

Understanding an ICD
An ICD consists of a pulse-generator box and a lead wire system that incorporates either one or two leads. The system shown here includes a ventricular lead wire and an atrial lead wire. Features of the generator and lead wires are detailed below.

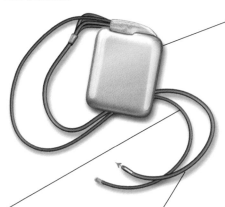

PULSE GENERATOR
- Is a small, battery-powered, programmable computer
- Monitors heart rate and rhythm
- Initiates the delivery of paced beats or defibrillatory shocks
- Stores information about the heart's activity before, during, and after an arrhythmia
- Tracks delivery and outcome of treatment
- Stores electrograms (similar to ECG strip when printed)
- Permits easy retrieval of all stored information

ATRIAL LEAD WIRE
- Is insulated
- Carries signals from the atrium to the pulse generator
- Delivers pacing impulses to the atrium

VENTRICULAR LEAD WIRE
- Is insulated
- Carries signals from the ventricle to the pulse generator
- Delivers electrical energy from the pulse generator to the ventricle

Implantable cardioverter-defibrillator placement

A specially trained cardiologist implants the pulse generator and lead wires in the cardiac catheterization laboratory with the patient under local anesthesia. Occasionally, a patient who requires other surgery, such as coronary artery bypass, may have the device implanted in the operating room.

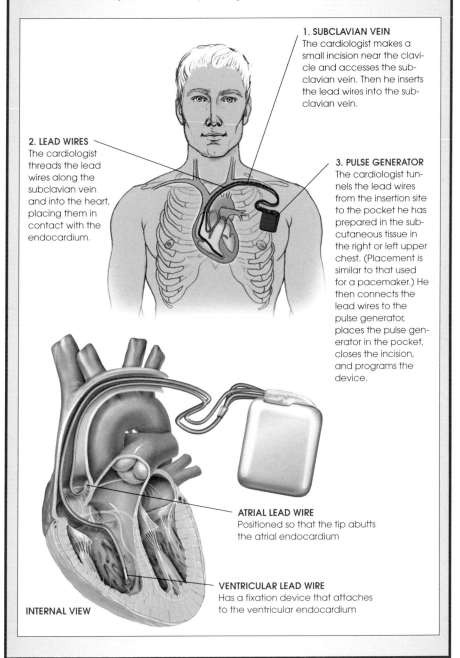

1. SUBCLAVIAN VEIN
The cardiologist makes a small incision near the clavicle and accesses the subclavian vein. Then he inserts the lead wires into the subclavian vein.

2. LEAD WIRES
The cardiologist threads the lead wires along the subclavian vein and into the heart, placing them in contact with the endocardium.

3. PULSE GENERATOR
The cardiologist tunnels the lead wires from the insertion site to the pocket he has prepared in the subcutaneous tissue in the right or left upper chest. (Placement is similar to that used for a pacemaker.) He then connects the lead wires to the pulse generator, places the pulse generator in the pocket, closes the incision, and programs the device.

ATRIAL LEAD WIRE
Positioned so that the tip abuts the atrial endocardium

VENTRICULAR LEAD WIRE
Has a fixation device that attaches to the ventricular endocardium

INTERNAL VIEW

Antiarrhythmic drugs and the action potential

Each class of antiarrhythmic drugs acts on a different phase of the cardiac action potential to alter the heart's electrophysiology.

Class I drugs

Class I drugs are sodium channel blockers that reduce the influx of sodium ions into the cell during phase 0 of the action potential.

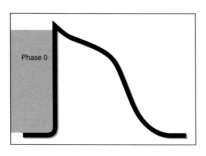

Class II drugs

Class II drugs inhibit adrenergic stimulation of cardiac tissue. They depress phase 4 spontaneous depolarization and slow sinoatrial node impulses.

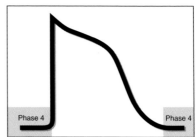

Class III drugs

Class III drugs are potassium channel blockers that prolong phase 3 of the action potential, thereby increasing repolarization and refractoriness.

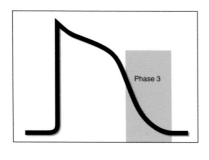

Class IV drugs

Class IV drugs inhibit calcium's slow influx into the cell during the action potential's plateau phase (phase 2). They depress phase 4 and lengthen phases 1 and 2.

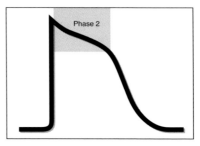

Recognizing RVH

The waveforms here show key electrocardiogram changes occurring in selected leads with right ventricular hypertrophy (RVH).

Normally, the R wave would progressively increase from V_1 to V_6. In RVH, the R wave gets progressively smaller from V_1 to V_6. In lead V_1, you'll note a tall R wave (see highlighted area). In lead V_6, the S wave is deepened (see highlighted area) and the amplitude of the S wave is equal to or greater than that of the R wave (see arrows).

LEAD V_1

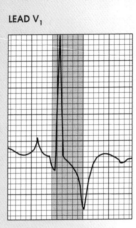

LEAD V_6

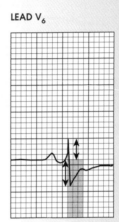

T wave: Inverted in V_1 and V_2
QT interval: Usually normal
Other: Right axis deviation may be present

Signs and symptoms

Signs and symptoms may be related to the underlying cause. With pulmonary hypertension and RVH, the patient may experience dizziness, shortness of breath, or syncope.

Interventions

Treatment focuses on management of the underlying disorder such as pulmonary hypertension.

LEFT VENTRICULAR HYPERTROPHY

In *left ventricular hypertrophy* (LVH), the left ventricular wall thickens. LVH usually results from conditions that cause chronic increases in pressure within the ventricle.

Causes

LVH may be caused by mitral insufficiency, cardiomyopathy, aortic stenosis or insufficiency, or systemic hypertension (the most common

Recognizing LVH

Left ventricular hypertrophy (LVH) can lead to heart failure or myocardial infarction. The rhythm strip shown here illustrates key electrocardiogram changes of LVH as they occur in selected leads: a large S wave (shaded area below left) in V_1 and a large R wave (shaded area below right) in V_5. If the depth (in mm) of the S wave in V_1 added to the height (in mm) of the R wave in V_5 is greater than 35 mm, then LVH is present.

LEAD V_1

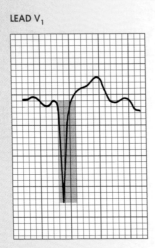

LEAD V_5

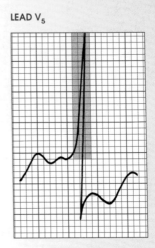

cause). LVH may lead to left-sided heart failure, which subsequently leads to increased left atrial pressure, pulmonary vascular congestion, and pulmonary arterial hypertension. LVH can decrease coronary artery perfusion, causing MI, or it can alter the papillary muscle, causing mitral insufficiency.

ECG characteristics

Rhythm: Atrial and ventricular rhythms normal

Rate: Atrial and ventricular rates normal

P wave: May be normal in size and configuration, or may reflect left atrial enlargement

PR interval: Normal

QRS complex: May be prolonged or widened with increased amplitude; increasing amplitude of R wave in leads I, aV_L, V_5, and V_6; S wave amplitude increasing in leads V_1 and V_2; LVH existing if depth of S wave in V_1 added to the height of R wave in V_5 appears greater than 35 mm (See *Recognizing LVH*.)

ST segment: Possibly depressed in the precordial leads when associated with T-wave inversion; this pattern known as *LVH with strain*

T wave: May be inverted in leads V_5 or V_6 depending on the degree of hypertrophy

QT interval: Usually normal

Other: Axis usually normal, but left axis deviation may be present

Signs and symptoms

Signs and symptoms are related to the underlying disorder.

Interventions

Treatment focuses on management of the underlying disorder such as hypertension.

9 *Tachycardias*

Tachycardia poses a serious threat because it can reduce cardiac output, triggering hemodynamic instability. As the ventricular rate rises above normal, the amount of time that blood can flow into the ventricles — known as *ventricular filling time* — shortens. Thus, less blood flows into the ventricles between contractions, causing less blood to be ejected with each contraction.

This reduction in the amount of blood ejected per contraction, known as *stroke volume*, doesn't automatically reduce cardiac output. Cardiac output — the amount of blood ejected per minute — is determined by both stroke volume and ventricular rate (cardiac output = stroke volume × ventricular rate). So although the heart is pumping less blood per contraction than normal, it's also contracting more times per minute than normal. The result: Cardiac output remains normal, but only if the ventricles are healthy, and only up to a point. If, for instance, the ventricular rate suddenly rises above 150 beats/minute, even a healthy heart may not be able to compensate. Cardiac output will fall, and hemodynamic instability will develop.

■ Mechanisms causing tachycardias

The mechanisms that cause tachycardias include altered automaticity, reentry, preexcitation syndromes, and triggered activity.

ALTERED AUTOMATICITY
Automaticity is a special characteristic of pacemaker cells that allows them to initiate electrical impulses spontaneously. If a cell's automaticity is increased or decreased, an arrhythmia can occur. Enhanced automaticity may result from drugs such as digoxin; from increased sympathetic stimulation from fever, exercise, and thyrotoxicosis; and from hypoxia. Tachycardia and premature beats are commonly caused by enhanced automaticity. Tachycardias that result from enhanced automaticity include sinus tachycardia, atrial tachycardia, and multifocal atrial tachycardia. Junctional tachycardia and ventricular tachycardia

How reentry develops

Normally, conduction occurs along a single pathway, so reentry can't occur. In some people, however, conduction occurs along two pathways — one fast and one slow. The speed and frequency of impulse conduction varies along those paths.

One pathway has a perfect surface for speed. The other pathway meanders through an obstacle course. An impulse starting off stays together until the pathways diverge.

Unidirectional conduction
When the pathways diverge, the impulses split up, as shown here. Half of the impulses take the fast pathway, and half struggle through obstacles on the slow pathway. The fast-pathway impulses reach the end point well

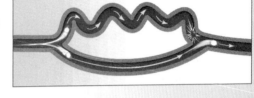

ahead of the slow-pathway impulses, which causes the slow-pathway impulses to stop moving and disperse.

Premature impulse
If an ectopic impulse reaches the pathways prematurely, the fast pathway isn't ready; it's still refractory from the previous conduction. In such cases, as shown here, the impulse takes the slow pathway, which can accept impulses more quickly.

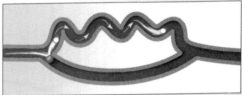

Reentry
When the impulses reach the bottom of the slow pathway, as shown here, one impulse splits off and heads to the end point. The others head back up the fast pathway. The impulse then continues around the circuit — down

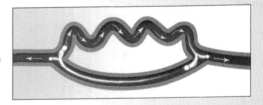

the slow pathway and up the fast pathway — repeatedly, sending one impulse each time to the end point and one back up to the starting point. That continuous looping of an impulse through the two pathways, known as *reentry*, can result in tachyarrhythmias.

may result from altered automaticity, but they usually result from a reentry mechanism.

REENTRY

Reentry occurs when cardiac tissue is activated two or more times by the same impulse. (See *How reentry develops.*) This repetition happens when

Conduction in WPW syndrome

Electrical impulses in the heart don't always follow normal conduction pathways. In preexcitation syndromes, electrical impulses enter the ventricles from the atria through an accessory pathway that bypasses the atrioventricular junction. Wolff-Parkinson-White (WPW) syndrome is a common type of preexcitation syndrome.

WPW syndrome commonly occurs in young children and in adults ages 20 to 35. It causes the PR interval to shorten and the QRS complex to lengthen as a result of a delta wave. Delta waves, which in WPW occur just before normal ventricular de-polarization, are produced as a result of the premature depolarization or preexcitation of a portion of the ventricles.

WPW is clinically significant because the accessory pathway — in this case, Kent's bundle — may result in paroxysmal tachyarrhythmias by reentry and rapid conduction mechanisms.

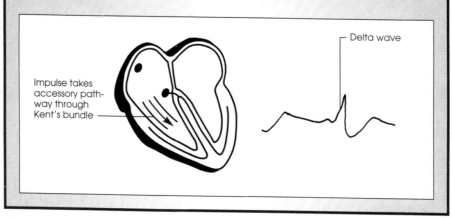

Delta wave

Impulse takes accessory pathway through Kent's bundle

conduction speed is slowed or when refractory periods for neighboring cells occur at different times. Impulses are delayed long enough that cells have time to repolarize, and the active impulse reenters the same area and produces another impulse. Reentry may result from ischemia, electrolyte imbalances, and drugs. Reentry may occur in young adults without heart disease, and atrioventricular (AV) nodal reentrant tachy-cardia is most commonly seen in these patients. Tachycardias that may result from a reentry mechanism include paroxysmal atrial tachycardia, atrial flutter, atrial fibrillation, junctional tachycardia, and ventricular tachycardia.

PREEXCITATION SYNDROME

Preexcitation syndrome, a form of reentry, is an early activation of the ventricles when the supraventricular impulse bypasses the AV node and activates the ventricles by way of a bypass tract or accessory pathway. Because the impulse doesn't pass through the AV node, no impulse delay results that normally would occur at the AV node, and the impulse reaches the ventricles sooner than it would through the normal conduction pathway. As a result, a rhythm with a dangerously fast rate occurs. Wolff-Parkinson-White (WPW) syndrome is a preexcitation syndrome that's commonly seen in young children and young adults. (See *Conduction in WPW syndrome.*)

TRIGGERED ACTIVITY

Pacemaker cells, when injured, may partially depolarize rather than fully depolarizing. Partial depolarization can lead to spontaneous or second-ary depolarization or repetitive ectopic firings, called *triggered activity.* The resultant depolarization is called *afterdepolarization.* Early after depolarization occurs before the cell is fully repolarized and can be caused by hypokalemia, drug toxicity, or slow pacing rates. If it occurs after the cell has been fully repolarized, it's called *delayed afterdepolariza-tion,* and may result from digoxin toxicity, hypercalcemia, or increased catecholamine release. Atrial tachycardia and ventricular tachycardia may result from this mechanism.

■ *Narrow-complex tachycardias*

With narrow-complex tachycardias, the duration of the QRS complex (and of ventricular depolarization) is within normal limits. The QRS complex is normal and termed "narrow" when compared with the wide QRS complex that characterizes wide-complex tachycardias.

   Narrow-complex tachycardias are also referred to as *supraventricular tachycardias (SVTs),* because the abnormal impulse originates above the ventricles. The impulse may begin in the sinoatrial (SA) node, the atria, or the AV junction, including the AV node and bundle of His. The impulse then travels through the heart's conduction system depolarizing both ventricles simultaneously, and producing a narrow QRS complex.

ECG CHARACTERISTICS

Narrow-complex tachycardias have a QRS complex with a normal dura-tion (0.06 to 0.10 second), indicating that the impulse originates above the ventricles and follows the normal conduction pathway. With narrow-complex tachycardia, however, the complexes will also be close together. Sometimes they're so close that only a single wave is visible between them. It may be difficult to distinguish the P wave from the preceding T wave, in which case the waves form a T-P configuration because the P wave is buried in the preceding T wave.

   The general electrocardiogram (ECG) characteristics of narrow-complex tachycardia are:
■ a ventricular rate greater than 100 beats/minute
■ a normal-width QRS complex
■ regular rhythm (for most rhythms except atrial fibrillation, atrial flut-ter, and multifocal arterial tachycardia [MAT]). (See *Identifying narrow-complex tachycardia,* page 158.)

Identifying narrow-complex tachycardia

The rhythm strip shown here illustrates narrow-complex tachycardia. Look for these distinguishing characteristics.

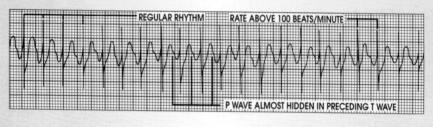

REGULAR RHYTHM   RATE ABOVE 100 BEATS/MINUTE

P WAVE ALMOST HIDDEN IN PRECEDING T WAVE

■ *Types of narrow-complex tachycardias*

Narrow-complex tachycardias are those arrhythmias that originate above the ventricles, in the SA node, atria, and AV junction. They have an accelerated rate and a narrow QRS complex. Types of narrow-complex tachycardias include sinus tachycardia, atrial tachycardia, atrial fibrillation, atrial flutter, multifocal atrial tachycardia, paroxysmal atrial tachycardia, WPW syndrome, and junctional tachycardia.

SINUS TACHYCARDIA

Sinus tachycardia is an acceleration of the firing of the SA node beyond its normal discharge rate, resulting in a heart rate of 100 to 160 beats/minute. Rates greater than 160 beats/minute may indicate ectopic focus. Persistent sinus tachycardia, especially with acute myocardial infarction (MI), may lead to ischemia and myocardial damage by raising oxygen requirements.

Sinus tachycardia may occur as a normal cardiac response to demand for increased oxygen during exercise, fever, stress, pain, and dehydration. It may also develop as a normal part of the inflammatory response after an MI. Other causes include such triggers as caffeine, nicotine, and alcohol; such medications as adrenergics, anticholinergics, antiarrhythmics, and digoxin; hypothyroidism or hyperthyroidism; and any other occurrence that decreases vagal tone and increases sympathetic tone. Generally treatment for sinus tachycardia is aimed at correcting the underlying cause. It's important to differentiate sinus tachycardia from other forms of SVT so that appropriate treatment measures will be initiated. (See *Identifying sinus tachycardia.*)

Identifying sinus tachycardia

The rhythm strip shown here illustrates sinus tachycardia. Look for these distinguishing characteristics.

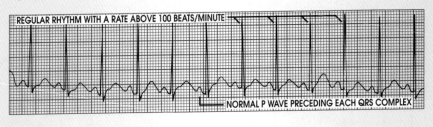

REGULAR RHYTHM WITH A RATE ABOVE 100 BEATS/MINUTE

NORMAL P WAVE PRECEDING EACH QRS COMPLEX

ATRIAL FIBRILLATION

Atrial fibrillation, sometimes called *A-fib*, is defined as chaotic, asynchronous, electrical activity in atrial tissue. It stems from a firing of a number of impulses in reentry pathways. Like atrial flutter, atrial fibrillation results in a loss of atrial kick. The ectopic impulses fire at a rate over 400 times/minute, causing the atria to quiver instead of contract.

The ventricles respond only to those impulses that make it through the AV node. On the ECG, atrial activity is no longer represented by P waves but by erratic baseline waves called *fibrillatory waves* or *f waves*. This rhythm may be either sustained or may occur in bursts. It can be preceded by or the result of premature atrial contractions (PACs).

A-fib may simply occur from aging. Other causes include chronic obstructive pulmonary disease, valvular disorders (especially mitral stenosis), hypertension, MI, coronary artery disease, heart failure, cardiomyopathy, pericarditis, rheumatic heart disease, thyrotoxicosis, cardiac surgery, and certain medications such as digoxin. Occasionally, it may result from increased sympathetic activity from exercise. (See *Identifying atrial fibrillation.*)

Identifying atrial fibrillation

The rhythm strip shown here illustrates atrial fibrillation. Look for these distinguishing characteristics.

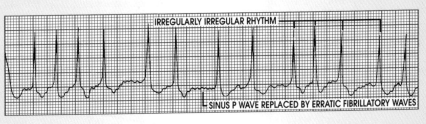

IRREGULARLY IRREGULAR RHYTHM

SINUS P WAVE REPLACED BY ERRATIC FIBRILLATORY WAVES

Identifying atrial flutter

Atrial flutter has a regular atrial rhythm with a rate of 250 to 400 beats/minute. Ventricular rate can vary, depending on the atrioventricular conduction pattern, although it's often regular. The P wave is sawtoothed and referred to as a *flutter wave.*

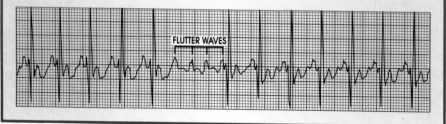

FLUTTER WAVES

 LEAD OF CHOICE Lead II or the leads that best show the fibrillatory waves are the optimal choices for monitoring the patient with atrial fibrillation.

ATRIAL FLUTTER

Atrial flutter is characterized by a rapid atrial rate. The ventricular rate varies depending on the degree of AV block. The rhythm originates in one atrial focus, resulting from circus reentry mechanism. On the ECG, the P waves lose their normal appearance due to the rapid atrial rate. The waves blend together in a sawtooth configuration called *flutter waves* (the hallmark characteristic of the rhythm). (See *Identifying atrial flutter.*)

The patient may develop an atrial rhythm that varies between a fibrillatory line and flutter waves. This variation is referred to as *atrial fibflutter.* The ventricular response is irregular. At times it may be difficult to distinguish atrial flutter from atrial fibrillation. (See *Distinguishing atrial flutter from atrial fibrillation.*)

The significance of atrial flutter depends on the extent to which the ventricular rate is accelerated. The faster this rate is, the more dangerous the arrhythmia is. Even a small rise in rate can cause angina, syncope, hypotension, heart failure, and pulmonary edema. Atrial flutter may be caused by acute or chronic cardiac disorders, mitral or tricuspid valve disorders, cor pulmonale, and cardiac inflammation such as pericarditis. Other causes include MI, digoxin toxicity, hyperthyroidism, alcoholism, and cardiac surgery.

 LEAD OF CHOICE Leads II and III are the best leads for monitoring the patient with atrial flutter. Lead aV_F on the 12-lead ECG is helpful in identifying flutter waves.

LOOK-ALIKES

Distinguishing atrial flutter from atrial fibrillation

It isn't uncommon to see atrial flutter that has an irregular pattern of impulse conduction to the ventricles. In some leads, this may be confused with atrial fibrillation.
Here's how to tell the two arrhythmias apart.

Atrial flutter
- Look for characteristic abnormal P waves that produce a sawtooth appearance, referred to as *flutter waves*, or *F waves*. These can best be identified in leads
I, II, and aV$_F$.
- Remember that the atrial rhythm is regular. You should be able to map the flutter
waves across the rhythm strip. While some flutter waves may occur within the QRS
or T waves, subsequent flutter waves will be visible and occur on time.

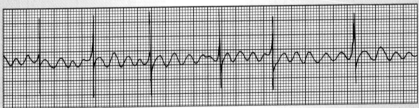

Atrial fibrillation
- Fibrillatory or f waves occur in an irregular pattern, making the atrial rhythm irregular.
- If you identify atrial activity that at times looks like flutter waves and seems to be
regular for a short time, and in other places the rhythm strip contains fibrillatory
waves, interpret the rhythm as atrial fibrillation. Coarse fibrillatory waves may intermittently look similar to the characteristic sawtooth appearance of flutter waves.

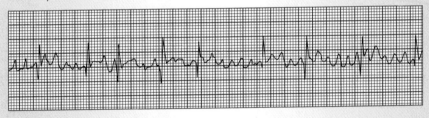

MULTIFOCAL ATRIAL TACHYCARDIA

In MAT, the atrial rhythm is ectopic, and the atrial rate ranges from 160
to 250 beats/minute. MAT results from an extremely rapid firing of multifocal ectopic sites. The distinguishing feature of the rhythm is that the
P-wave configuration varies and there are at least three different P-wave
shapes. (See *Identifying MAT*, page 162.) The variation in P-wave configuration and also the irregular rhythm is a result of the impulse shifting

Identifying MAT

In multifocal atrial tachycardia (MAT), atrial tachycardia occurs with numerous atrial foci firing intermittently. MAT produces varying P waves on the strip and occurs most commonly in patients with chronic pulmonary disease. The irregular baseline shown below is caused by movement of the chest wall. Look for these distinguishing characteristics.

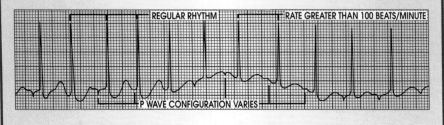

from the SA node to the atria and the AV junction. Because the rhythm is irregular, it may be difficult to distinguish from atrial fibrillation. (See *Distinguishing atrial fibrillation from MAT.*) Very rare in healthy individuals, MAT is usually found in acutely ill patients with pulmonary disease (such as chronic obstructive pulmonary disease), elevated atrial pressures, and heart failure. It may also result from MI, theophylline toxicity, and hypokalemia.

 LEAD OF CHOICE Leads II, V_1, and V_6, or the modified leads MCL_1 and MCL_6, are the best leads for monitoring the patient with MAT.

PAROXYSMAL ATRIAL TACHYCARDIA

Paroxysmal atrial tachycardia (PAT) arises suddenly; it's a type of paroxysmal supraventricular tachycardia. The hallmark of the rhythm is that it starts and stops suddenly. PAT may be benign when it occurs in a healthy person, unless it is sustained and results in hemodynamic instability. It results from a reentry mechanism. It may be caused by digoxin toxicity, MI, congenital heart disease, and cardiomyopathy. In healthy individuals, PAT may be caused by physical or psychological stress, hypoxia, hypokalemia or other electrolyte disturbances, excessive use of caffeine or other stimulants, and marijuana use. (See *Identifying PAT,* page 164.)

 LEAD OF CHOICE Leads II, V_1, and V_6, or the modified leads MCL_1 and MCL_6, are the best leads for monitoring the patient with PAT.

WOLFF-PARKINSON-WHITE SYNDROME

WPW syndrome, a preexcitation syndrome, occurs when an anomalous atrial bypass tract (bundle of Kent) develops outside the AV junction,

LOOK-ALIKES

Distinguishing atrial fibrillation from MAT

To help you determine whether a rhythm is atrial fibrillation or the similar multifocal atrial tachycardia (MAT), focus on the presence of P waves as well as the atrial and ventricular rhythms. You may find it helpful to look at a longer (greater than 6 seconds) rhythm strip.

Atrial fibrillation
- Carefully look for discernible P waves before each QRS complex.
- If you can't clearly identify P waves, and fibrillatory waves, appear in the place of P waves, then the rhythm is probably atrial fibrillation.
- Carefully look at the rhythm, focusing on the R-R intervals. Remember that one of the hallmarks of atrial fibrillation is an irregularly irregular rhythm.

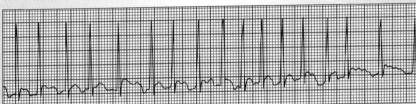

MAT
- P waves are present in MAT. Keep in mind, though, that the shape of the P waves will vary, with at least three different P-wave shapes visible in a single rhythm strip.
- You should be able to see most, if not all, of the various P-wave shapes repeat.
- Although the atrial and ventricular rhythms are irregular, the irregularity generally isn't as pronounced as it is in atrial fibrillation.

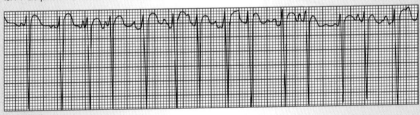

connecting the atria and the ventricles. This accessory pathway can conduct impulses either to the ventricles or the atria. With retrograde conduction, reentry can arise, resulting in a reentrant tachycardia.

Usually WPW syndrome is considered insignificant if tachycardia doesn't occur or if the patient has no associated cardiac disease. When tachycardia does occur in WPW syndrome, decreased cardiac output may develop.

Identifying PAT

A type of paroxysmal supraventricular tachycardia, paroxysmal atrial tachycardia (PAT) features brief periods of tachycardia that alternate with periods of normal sinus rhythm. It starts and stops suddenly as a result of rapid firing of an ectopic focus. PAT commonly follows frequent premature atrial contractions (PACs), one of which initiates the tachycardia. Look for these distinguishing characteristics.

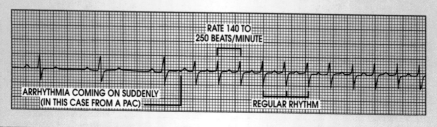

RATE 140 TO 250 BEATS/MINUTE

ARRHYTHMIA COMING ON SUDDENLY (IN THIS CASE FROM A PAC)

REGULAR RHYTHM

Congenital in origin, WPW syndrome manifests predominately in young children and in adults ages 20 to 35. (See *Identifying WPW syndrome*.)

ATRIOVENTRICULAR NODAL REENTRY TACHYCARDIA

AV nodal reentry tachycardia (AVNRT) is the most common type of narrow complex tachycardia and results from a reentry mechanism. A reentry circuit is set up in the AV node with two pathways, a slow pathway with a shorter refractory period and a fast pathway with a longer refractory period. The rhythm starts and stops suddenly and is usually initiated by a PAC. The PAC finds the fast pathway refractory and is conducted down the slow pathway, where it travels simultaneously into the ventricles and up the fast pathway to the atria and establishes a reentry circuit, which causes repeated, simultaneous stimulation of the atria and ventricles.

Identifying WPW syndrome

The hallmark of Wolff-Parkinson-White (WPW) syndrome is the delta wave, which is evident as a slurred wave at the beginning of the QRS complex and short PR interval.

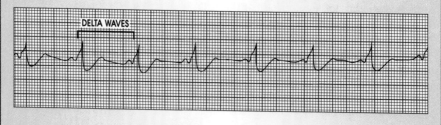

DELTA WAVES

Identifying AVNRT

Leads II, III, and aV_F show the characteristic findings of atrioventricular nodal reentry tachycardia (AVNRT). Note the retrograde P waves appearing immediately after the QRS complexes.

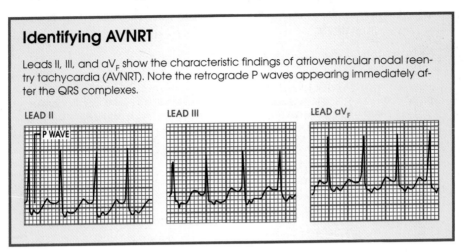

AVNRT commonly occurs in young adults without heart disease. It may occur in patients with preexisting heart disease, and if the heart rate exceeds 200 beats/minute, it may cause a decrease in cardiac output. (See *Identifying AVNRT.*)

■ *Types of wide-complex tachycardias*

Wide-complex tachycardias are arrhythmias that involve an accelerated heart rate and a wide QRS complex. In this type of tachycardia, an impulse originates in one of the ventricles and depolarizes it first. The impulse is then conducted to the other ventricle and depolarizes it. This delayed, sequential (rather than simultaneous) depolarization of the ventricles produces the wide QRS complex. Types of wide-complex tachycardia include monomorphic ventricular tachycardia, polymorphic ventricular tachycardia, torsades de pointes, and supraventricular rhythms with an intraventricular conduction abnormality or bundle-branch block.

Most supraventricular rhythms reach the ventricles simultaneously by way of the bundle branches and thus produce a narrow–QRS-complex tachycardia. But when the patient has a pathologic bundle-branch block, the supraventricular impulse will reach one ventricle first, then the other. Such sequential depolarization also occurs when the supraventricular impulse finds one of the bundle branches refractory. In either case, the delayed ventricular depolarization produces a wide QRS complex that may be difficult to distinguish from ventricular tachycardia (VT). (See *Distinguishing VT from SVT,* pages 166 and 167.)

MONOMORPHIC VENTRICULAR TACHYCARDIA

Monomorphic VT is the most common form of ventricular tachycardia. In this life-threatening arrhythmia, all of the QRS complexes are of the same morphology, indicating that they all originate from the same loca-

LOOK-ALIKES

Distinguishing VT from SVT

Differentiating ventricular tachycardia (VT) from supraventricular tachycardia (SVT) with aberrancy is difficult. However, careful assessment of a 12-lead electrocardiogram or rhythm strip can help you distinguish these arrhythmias with 90% accuracy. Begin by looking at the deflection to determine if it's negative or positive. Then use the illustrations shown here to guide your assessment.

Negative deflection
If the QRS complex is wide and the deflection is mostly negative in lead V₁ or MCL₁, use these illustrations to make your assessment.

Ventricular tachycardia
If the QRS complex has an R wave of 0.04 second or more, a slurred S (shown below, shaded), or a notched S on the downstroke (shown in inset below), suspect VT.

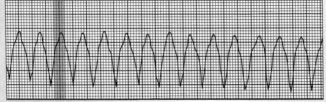 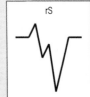

Supraventricular tachycardia
If the QRS complex has an R wave of 0.04 second or more and a swift, straight S on the downstroke (shown below, shaded, and in inset below), suspect SVT with aberrancy.

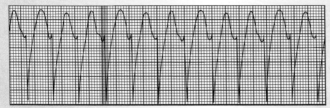 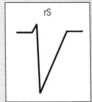

Positive deflection
If the QRS complex is wide and the deflection is mostly positive in lead V₁ or MCL₁, use these illustrations to make your assessment.

Ventricular tachycardia
If the QRS complex is biphasic, suspect VT (shown in inset below).

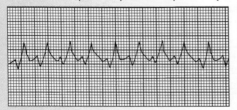 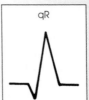 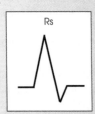

Distinguishing VT from SVT *(continued)*

Supraventricular tachycardia

If the beat is triphasic, similar to a right bundle-branch block, suspect SVT with aberrancy (shown in inset below).

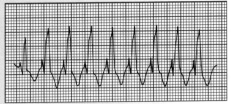

rR

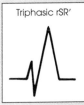

Triphasic rSR'

Other verification

Another way to distinguish VT from SVT is if the complex is wide and mostly positive in deflection in lead V_1 or MCL_1.

If the QRS complex is tall and shaped like rabbit ears, with the left peak taller than the right, suspect VT.

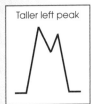

Taller left peak

If the QRS complex is monophasic, suspect VT.

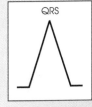

QRS

If you still have trouble differentiating the rhythm, look at lead V_6 or MCL_6.

If the S wave is larger than the R wave, suspect VT.

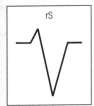

rS

If a Q wave is present, suspect VT.

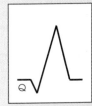

Q

Additional criteria

Other criteria can also help you differentiate VT from SVT with aberrancy:
- A QRS complex that exceeds 0.14 second suggests VT.
- A regular, wide, complex rhythm suggests VT.
- Concordant V leads (the QRS complex either mainly positive or mainly negative in all V leads) suggest VT.
- Atrioventricular dissociation suggests VT.

tion in the ventricles. Three or more premature ventricular contractions (PVCs) occur in succession at a rate of more than 100 beats/minute. The arrhythmia may be paroxysmal or sustained. The QRS complex duration exceeds 0.12 second with a wide, bizarre appearance; some complexes have increased amptitude. Because atrial and ventricular activity are dissociated and ventricular filling time is short, cardiac output may drop

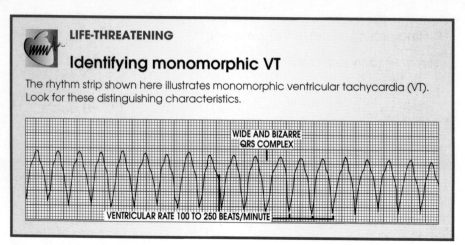

LIFE-THREATENING

Identifying monomorphic VT

The rhythm strip shown here illustrates monomorphic ventricular tachycardia (VT). Look for these distinguishing characteristics.

sharply. Monomorphic VT may lead to ventricular fibrillation. (See *Identifying monomorphic VT.*)

Monomorphic VT is usually caused by myocardial irritability and circuit reentry and may be precipitated by a PVC that occurs in the vulnerable period of ventricular repolarization (R-on-T phenomenon). Other causes include acute MI, cardiomyopathy, coronary artery disease (CAD), drug toxicity, electrolyte imbalance, heart failure, mitral valve prolapse, pulmonary embolism, and rheumatic heart disease.

 LEAD OF CHOICE Leads V_1 and V_6, or the modified leads MCL_1 and MCL_6, are the best leads for monitoring the patient with VT.

POLYMORPHIC VENTRICULAR TACHYCARDIA

Polymorphic VT is a form of VT in which the QRS complex morphology is unstable and continually varies because the site of origin changes

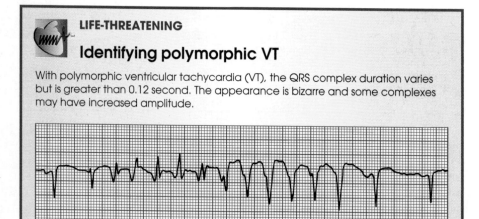

LIFE-THREATENING

Identifying polymorphic VT

With polymorphic ventricular tachycardia (VT), the QRS complex duration varies but is greater than 0.12 second. The appearance is bizarre and some complexes may have increased amplitude.

LIFE-THREATENING

Identifying TdP

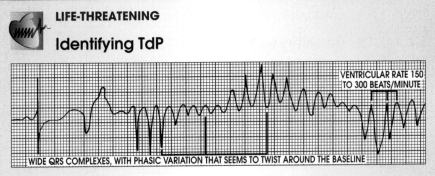

VENTRICULAR RATE 150 TO 300 BEATS/MINUTE

WIDE QRS COMPLEXES, WITH PHASIC VARIATION THAT SEEMS TO TWIST AROUND THE BASELINE

Torsades de pointes (TdP), which means "twisting of the points," is a special form of polymorphic ventricular tachycardia. The hallmark characteristics of this rhythm, shown above, are QRS complexes that rotate about the baseline, deflecting downward and upward for several beats.

The rate is 150 to 300 beats/minute, usually with an irregular rhythm, and the QRS complexes are wide with changing amplitude. The P wave is usually absent.

Paroxysmal rhythm

TdP may be paroxysmal, starting and stopping suddenly, and may deteriorate into ventricular fibrillation. It should be considered when ventricular tachycardia doesn't respond to antiarrhythmic therapy or other treatments.

Reversible causes

The cause of TdP is usually reversible. The most common causes are drugs that lengthen the QT interval, such as amiodarone, ibutilide, erythromycin, haloperidol, droperidol, and sotalol. Other causes include myocardial ischemia and electrolyte abnormalities such as hypokalemia, hypomagnesemia, and hypocalcemia.

Mechanical overdrive pacing

TdP is treated by correcting the underlying cause, especially if the cause is related to specific drug therapy. The physician may order mechanical overdrive pacing, which overrides the ventricular rate and breaks the triggered mechanism for the arrhythmia. Magnesium sulfate may also be effective. Electrical cardioversion may be used when TdP doesn't respond to other treatment.

throughout the ventricle. The QT interval is within normal limits when the patient is in normal sinus rhythm, unlike with torsades de pointes, in which the QT interval is prolonged. Polymorphic VT is associated with a poorer prognosis than that of monomorphic VT. Possible causes of polymorphic VT include MI and CAD. The QRS complex duration varies but is greater than 0.12 second with a bizarre appearance; some complexes have increased amplitude. (See *Identifying polymorphic VT.*)

TORSADES DE POINTES

A life-threatening arrhythmia, torsades de pointes (TdP) is a polymorphic VT characterized by a prolonged QT interval and QRS polarity that seems to spiral around the isoelectric line. Any condition that causes a prolonged QT interval can also cause TdP.

LOOK-ALIKES

Distinguishing ventricular flutter from TdP

Torsades de pointes (TdP) is a variant form of ventricular tachycardia, with a rapid ventricular rate that varies between 250 and 300 beats/minute. It's characterized by QRS complexes that gradually change back and forth, with the amplitude of each successive complex gradually increasing and decreasing. This movement results in an overall outline of the rhythm commonly described as *spindle-shaped*.

Ventricular flutter, although rarely recognized, results from the rapid, regular, repetitive beating of the ventricles. It's produced by a single ventricular focus firing at a rapid rate of 250 to 350 beats/minute. The hallmark of ventricular flutter is its smooth sine-wave appearance.

The illustrations shown here highlight key differences between the two arrhythmias.

VENTRICULAR FLUTTER
- Smooth, sine-wave appearance

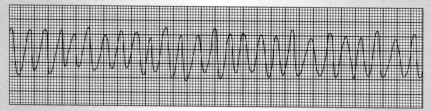

TORSADES DE POINTES
- Spindle-shaped appearance

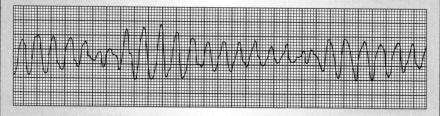

Although a regular rhythm may resume spontaneously, TdP usually degenerates to ventricular fibrillation. It may be difficult to distinguish TdP from ventricular flutter. (See *Identifying TdP*, page 169, and *Distinguishing ventricular flutter from TdP*.)

Causes of TdP include AV block, drug toxicity (particularly sotalol, quinidine, procainamide, and related antiarrhythmics such as disopyramide). Other causes include electrolyte imbalance, hereditary QT prolongation, myocardial ischemia, Prinzmetal's angina, psychotropic drugs and SA disease that results in profound tachycardia. Identification of patients at risk for TdP may help prevent the arrhythmia. It's important to

Interpreting QTc measurements

Calculating the QT

The QT interval measures the time needed for the ventricular depolarization-repolarization cycle. The measurement begins at the beginning of the QRS complex and extends to the end of the T wave.

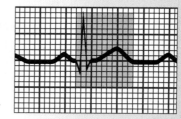

The formula that can be used to determine the normal QT interval is:

- Normal QT = 0.39 (square root of the R-R interval (in seconds)) ±10%
- Normal values are 0.36 to 0.44 second but can be affected by age, sex, and heart rate.

The QT interval can help identify life-threatening problems. A useful way to identify a normal QT interval is to note that the QT interval should be less than half the preceding R-R interval; however, this formula only works for heart rates between 65 and 90 beats/minute.

Calculating the QTc

QTc stands for *QT corrected*. A mathematical formula known as *Bazett's formula* was devised to correct the QT interval for the patient's heart rate.

The formula that can be used to determine QTc is:

- QTc = QT measured / square root of the R-R interval (in seconds)
- Normal values are 0.39 second in males and 0.41 second in females.

Using the QTc

Calculating the QTc and comparing it to the normal value can help determine prolonged ventricular depolarization-repolarization. A prolonged QT or QTc suggests abnormal effects on the myocardium.

calculate the QTc (which stands for *QT corrected*) interval to identify patients with a prolonged QT interval and a history of prolonged QT syndrome. (See *Interpreting QTc measurements,* and *Understanding the prolonged QT syndrome,* page 172.)

Understanding the prolonged QT syndrome.

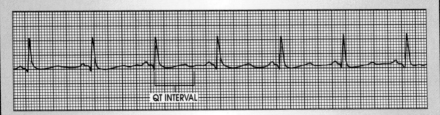

QT INTERVAL

The QT interval represents ventricular depolarization (electrical activation) and repolarization (electrical recovery of ventricular myocardial cells). When this interval becomes prolonged, it provides an opportunity for the development of torsades de pointes (TdP).

Electrocardiogram characteristics

Rhythm: Atrial and ventricular rhythms regular
Rate: Atrial and ventricular rates within normal limits
P wave: Normal size and configuration
PR interval: Within normal limits
QRS complex: Within normal limits, unless associated interventricular conduction delay present
T wave: Within normal limits
QT interval: More than half the R-R interval
Other: Duration of the QT interval dependent on the heart rate (A QT interval less than half the distance between consecutive R waves (the R-R interval) is normal. It becomes longer with slow heart rates and shorter with rapid heart rates. The upper normal QT interval for a heart rate of 60 beats/minute shouldn't exceed 0.43 second.)

Causes
■ Electrolyte imbalances
■ Drugs, including phenothiazines, probucol, erythromycin, thiazides, and antiarrhythmics such as quinidine, procainamide, disopyramide, flecainide, amiodarone, sotalol, and bepridil

■ Rare congenital syndromes, such as Jervell and Lange-Nielsen syndromes
■ Miscellaneous causes, such as myocardial ischemia, subarachnoid hemorrhage, ruptured cerebral aneurysm, streptococcal meningitis, hypothermia, and liquid protein diets

Signs and symptoms
■ No specific signs and symptoms associated with prolonged QT syndrome (However, a life-threatening arrhythmia may be accompanied by feelings of impending anxiety, decreased mentation, or loss of consciousness.)
■ Possibly signs and symptoms of low cardiac output

Interventions
■ For prolonged QT interval, slow infusions of I.V. potassium are used to raise potassium levels to high normal.
■ I.V. magnesium may be used to suppress TdP.
■ Isoproterenol or ventricular pacing may be used to increase heart rate and shorten the QT interval.
■ Discontinue any drugs that may be contributing to the patient's QT prolongation.
■ Revascularization by angioplasty or atherectomy may improve or reverse ischemia.
■ Electrical cardioversion or defibrillation may be performed, although they may only be transiently effective in terminating TdP.

10 *Electrolyte disturbances*

This chapter reviews electrocardiogram (ECG) characteristics associated with electrolyte disturbances.

Rhythm strips of patients with electrolyte disturbances, such as hyperkalemia, hypokalemia, hypercalcemia, and hypocalcemia, commonly show distinctive patterns. By recognizing some of these variations early, you may be able to identify and treat potentially dangerous conditions before they become serious.

Keep in mind, however, that the patient's ECG is only part of the clinical picture. Additional information, such as the patient's medical history, findings on physical examination, and additional diagnostic studies, will be necessary to confirm an initial diagnosis based on ECG analysis.

■ *Electrolyte disturbances*

Potassium and calcium ions play a major role in the electrical activity of the heart. *Depolarization* results from the exchange of these ions across the cell membrane. Changes in ion concentration can affect the heart's electrical activity and, as a result, the patient's ECG. This section examines ECG effects from high and low potassium and calcium levels.

HYPERKALEMIA
Potassium, the most plentiful intracellular cation (positively charged electrolyte), contributes to many important cellular functions. Most of the body's potassium content is located in the cells. The intracellular fluid (ICF) concentration of potassium is 150 to 160 mEq/L; the extracellular fluid (ECF) concentration, 3.5 to 4.5 mEq/L. Many symptoms associated with potassium imbalance result from changes in this ratio of ICF to ECF potassium concentration. Hyperkalemia is generally defined as an elevation of serum potassium above 5 mEq/L.

Causes
■ An increased intake of potassium, including excessive dietary intake and I.V. administration of penicillin G, potassium supplements, or banked whole blood

ECG effects of hyperkalemia

The classic and most striking electrocardiogram (ECG) feature of hyperkalemia is tall, peaked T waves. This rhythm strip shows a typical peaked T wave (shaded area).

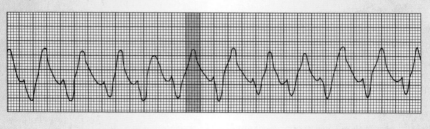

- A shift of potassium from ICF to ECF occurring with changes in cell membrane permeability or damage, including extensive surgery, burns, massive crush injuries, cell hypoxia, acidosis, and insulin deficiency
- Decreased renal excretion, including renal failure, decreased production and secretion of aldosterone, Addison's disease, and use of potassium-sparing diuretics

Clinical significance

When extracellular potassium concentrations increase without a significant change in intracellular potassium concentrations, the cell becomes less negative, or partially depolarized, and the resting cell membrane potential decreases. Mild elevations in extracellular potassium result in cells that repolarize faster and are more irritable.

 RED FLAG More critical elevations in extracellular potassium result in an inability of cells to repolarize and respond to electrical stimuli. Cardiac standstill, or *asystole,* is the most serious consequence of severe hyperkalemia.

ECG characteristics

Rhythm: Atrial and ventricular rhythms regular
Rate: Atrial and ventricular rates within normal limits
P wave: Low amplitude in mild hyperkalemia; wide and flattened P wave in moderate hyperkalemia; possible indiscernible P wave in severe hyperkalemia
PR interval: Normal or prolonged; not measurable if P wave can't be detected
QRS complex: Widened because ventricular depolarization takes longer
ST segment: May be elevated in severe hyperkalemia
T wave: Tall, peaked; the classic and most striking feature of hyperkalemia
QT interval: Shortened
Other: Intraventricular conduction disturbances commonly occurring
(See *ECG effects of hyperkalemia.*)

Signs and symptoms

Mild hyperkalemia may cause neuromuscular irritability, including restlessness, intestinal cramping, diarrhea, and tingling lips and fingers. Severe hyperkalemia may cause loss of muscle tone, muscle weakness, and paralysis.

Interventions

Treatment depends upon the severity of hyperkalemia and the patient's signs and symptoms. The underlying cause must be identified and the extracellular potassium concentration brought back to normal. Drug therapy to normalize potassium levels includes calcium gluconate to decrease neuromuscular irritability, insulin and glucose to facilitate the entry of potassium into the cell, and sodium bicarbonate to correct metabolic acidosis.

Oral or rectal administration of cation exchange resins, such as sodium polystyrene sulfonate, may be used to exchange sodium for potassium in the intestine. In the instance of renal failure or severe hyperkalemia, dialysis may be necessary to remove excess potassium. The patient's serum potassium levels should be monitored closely until they return to normal, and arrhythmias should be identified and managed appropriately.

HYPOKALEMIA

Hypokalemia, or potassium deficiency, occurs when the ECF concentration of potassium drops below 3.5 mEq/L, usually indicating a loss of total body potassium. The concentration of ECF potassium is so small that even minor changes in ECF potassium affect resting membrane potential.

Causes

- Increased loss of body potassium, increased entry of potassium into cells, and reduced potassium intake (Shifts in potassium from the extracellular space to the intracellular space may be caused by alkalosis, especially respiratory alkalosis. Intracellular uptake of potassium is also increased by catecholamines.)
- Although rare, dietary deficiency in elderly patients
- Alcoholism and anorexia nervosa
- GI and renal disorders (most commonly cause potassium loss from body stores) GI losses of potassium are associated with laxative abuse, intestinal fistulae or drainage tubes, diarrhea, vomiting, and continuous nasogastric drainage. Renal loss of potassium is related to increased secretion of potassium by the distal tubule. Diuretics, a low serum magnesium concentration, and excessive aldosterone secretion may cause urinary loss of potassium.
- Several antibiotics, including gentamicin and amphotericin B

ECG effects of hypokalemia

As the serum potassium concentration drops, the T wave becomes flat and a U wave appears (shaded area). This rhythm strip shows typical electrocardiogram (ECG) effects of hypokalemia.

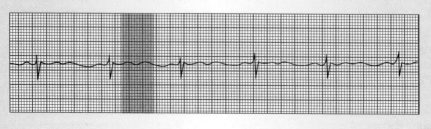

Clinical significance

When extracellular potassium levels decrease rapidly and intracellular potassium concentration doesn't change, the resting membrane potential becomes more negative and the cell membrane becomes hyperpolarized. The cardiac effects of hypokalemia are related to these changes in membrane excitability. Ventricular repolarization is delayed because potassium contributes to the repolarization phase of the action potential.

 RED FLAG Hypokalemia can cause dangerous ventricular arrhythmias and increases the risk of digoxin toxicity.

ECG characteristics

Rhythm: Atrial and ventricular rhythms regular
Rate: Atrial and ventricular rates within normal limits
P wave: Usually normal size and configuration, but may become peaked in severe hypokalemia
PR interval: May be prolonged
QRS complex: Within normal limits or possibly widened; prolonged in severe hypokalemia
QT interval: Usually indiscernible as the T wave flattens
ST segment: Depressed
T wave: Decreased amplitude (The T wave becomes flat as the potassium level drops. In severe hypokalemia, it flattens completely and may become inverted. The T wave may also fuse with an increasingly prominent U wave.)
Other: Increased amplitude of U wave, becoming more prominent as hypokalemia worsens, and fusing with T wave (See *ECG effects of hypokalemia.*)

Signs and symptoms

The most common symptoms of hypokalemia are caused by neuromuscular and cardiac effects, including smooth muscle atony, skeletal mus-

cle weakness, and cardiac arrhythmias. Loss of smooth muscle tone results in constipation, intestinal distention, nausea, vomiting, anorexia,
and paralytic ileus.

 RED FLAG In hypokalemia, skeletal muscle weakness occurs
first in the larger muscles of the arms and legs and eventually
affects the diaphragm, causing respiratory arrest.

Cardiac effects of hypokalemia include arrhythmias, such as bradycardia, atrioventricular (AV) block, and ventricular arrhythmias. Delayed
depolarization results in characteristic changes on the ECG.

Interventions
The underlying causes of hypokalemia should be identified and corrected. Acid-base imbalances should be corrected, potassium losses replaced, and further losses prevented. Encourage intake of foods and flu-
ids rich in potassium. Oral or I.V. potassium supplements may be administered. The patient's serum potassium levels should be monitored
closely until they return to normal, and cardiac arrhythmias should be
identified and managed appropriately.

HYPERCALCEMIA
Most of the body's calcium stores (99%) are located in bone. The remain-
der is found in the plasma and body cells. Approximately 50% of plasma
calcium is bound to plasma proteins. About 40% is found in the ionized
or free form.

Calcium plays an important role in myocardial contractility. Ionized
calcium is more important than plasma-bound calcium in physiologic
functions. Hypercalcemia is usually defined as a serum calcium concentration greater than 10.5 mg/dl.

Causes
- Excess vitamin D intake
- Bone metastasis and calcium resorption associated with cancers of
the breast, prostate, and cervix
- Hyperparathyroidism
- Sarcoidosis
- Parathyroid hormone–producing tumors

Clinical significance
In hypercalcemia, calcium is found inside cells in greater abundance
than normal. The cell membrane becomes refractory to depolarization
as a result of a more positive action potential. This loss of cell membrane
excitability causes many of the cardiac symptoms seen in patients with
hypercalcemia.

Both ventricular depolarization and repolarization are accelerated.
The patient may experience bradyarrhythmias and varying degrees of AV
block.

ECG effects of hypercalcemia

Increased serum concentrations of calcium cause shortening of the QT interval as shown (shaded area) in this electrocardiogram (ECG) rhythm strip.

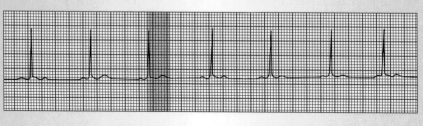

ECG characteristics

Rhythm: Atrial and ventricular rhythms regular
Rate: Atrial and ventricular rates within normal limits, but bradycardia can occur
P wave: Normal size and configuration
PR interval: May be prolonged
QRS complex: Within normal limits, but may be prolonged
QT interval: Shortened
ST segment: Shortened
T wave: Normal size and configuration; may be depressed
Other: None (See *ECG effects of hypercalcemia.*)

Signs and symptoms

Common signs and symptoms of hypercalcemia include anorexia, nausea, constipation, lethargy, fatigue, and weakness. Behavioral changes may also occur. Renal calculi may form as precipitates of calcium salts, and impaired renal function commonly occurs. A reciprocal decrease in serum phosphate levels often accompanies elevated levels of serum calcium.

Interventions

Treatment of hypercalcemia focuses on identifying and managing the underlying cause and is guided by the severity of the patient's symptoms. The administration of oral phosphate is usually effective as long as renal function is normal. In more critical situations, I.V. administration of large volumes of normal saline solution may enhance renal excretion of calcium. Patients in renal failure may need dialysis. Corticosteroids and calcitonin may be used to treat hypercalcemia.

HYPOCALCEMIA

Hypocalcemia occurs when the serum calcium level is below 8.5 mg/dl.

Causes

- Decreases in parathyroid hormone and vitamin D, inadequate intestinal absorption, blood administration, or deposition of ionized calcium into soft tissue or bone
- Inadequate dietary intake of green, leafy vegetables or dairy products resulting in a nutritional deficiency of calcium
- Excessive dietary intake of phosphorus that binds with calcium and prevents calcium absorption
- Citrate solution, used in storing whole blood, binding with calcium
- Pancreatitis, which decreases ionized calcium, and neoplastic bone metastases, which decrease serum calcium levels
- Decreased intestinal absorption of calcium caused by vitamin D deficiency, either from inadequate vitamin D intake or insufficient exposure to sunlight
- Malabsorption of fats, removal of the parathyroid glands, metabolic or respiratory alkalosis, and hypoalbuminemia

Clinical significance

Hypocalcemia causes an increase in neuromuscular excitability. Partial depolarization of nerves and muscle cells result from a decrease in threshold potential. As a result, a smaller stimulus is needed to initiate an action potential. Characteristic ECG changes are a result of prolonged ventricular depolarization and decreased cardiac contractility.

ECG characteristics

Rhythm: Atrial and ventricular rhythms regular
Rate: Atrial and ventricular rates within normal limits
P wave: Normal size and configuration
PR interval: Within normal limits
QRS complex: Within normal limits
QT interval: Prolonged
ST segment: Prolonged
T wave: Normal size and configuration, but may become flat or inverted
Other: None (See *ECG effects of hypocalcemia,* page 180.)

Signs and symptoms

Signs and symptoms of hypocalcemia include hyperreflexia, carpopedal spasm, confusion, and circumoral and digital paresthesia. Hyperactive bowel sounds and intestinal cramping may also occur.

 RED FLAG In hypocalcemia, severe symptoms include tetany, seizures, respiratory arrest, and death. Clinical signs indicating hypocalcemia include Trousseau's sign and Chvostek's sign.

ECG effects of hypocalcemia

Decreased serum concentrations of calcium prolong the QT interval, as shown (shaded area) in this electrocardiogram (ECG) rhythm strip.

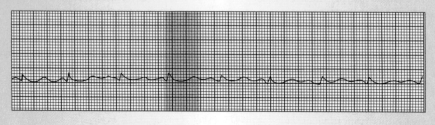

Interventions

Treatment should focus on identifying and managing the underlying causes of hypocalcemia. Severe signs and symptoms require emergency treatment with I.V. calcium gluconate. Serum calcium levels should be monitored and oral calcium replacement initiated when possible. Cardiac arrhythmias need to be identified and managed appropriately. Long-term management of hypocalcemia includes decreasing phosphate intake.

Part IV
Understanding the effects of treatment

11 *Pharmacologic treatment for arrhythmias*

■ *Cardiac drugs*

Almost half a million U.S. residents die each year from cardiac arrhythmias; countless others experience symptoms and lifestyle modifications. Along with other treatments, cardiac drugs can help alleviate symptoms, control heart rate and rhythm, decrease preload and afterload, and prolong life.

UNDERSTANDING ANTIARRHYTHMICS

Antiarrhythmics affect the movement of ions across the cell membrane and alter the electrophysiology of the cardiac cell. These drugs are classified according to their effect on the cell's electrical activity (*action potential*) and their mechanism of action. Because the drugs can cause changes in the myocardial action potential, characteristic electrocardiogram (ECG) changes can occur. (See *Antiarrhythmic drugs and the action potential*.)

The classification system divides antiarrhythmic drugs into four major classes based on their dominant mechanism of action: class I, class II, class III, and class IV. Class I antiarrhythmics are further divided into class IA, class IB, and class IC.

Certain antiarrhythmics can't be classified specifically into one group. For example, sotalol possesses characteristics of both class II and class III drugs. Still other drugs, such as adenosine, atropine, digoxin, epinephrine, vasopressin, and magnesium, don't fit into the classification system at all. Despite its limitations, the classification system is helpful in understanding how antiarrhythmics prevent and treat arrhythmias.

This chapter reviews ECG changes that result when patients take therapeutic doses of antiarrhythmics (separated by classification) and digoxin. When drug levels are toxic, ECG changes are typically exaggerated.

182

Antiarrhythmic drugs and the action potential

Each class of antiarrhythmic drugs acts on a different phase of the action potential and alters the heart's electrophysiology. Below is a summary of the four classes of antiarrhythmics and how each class affects the action potential.

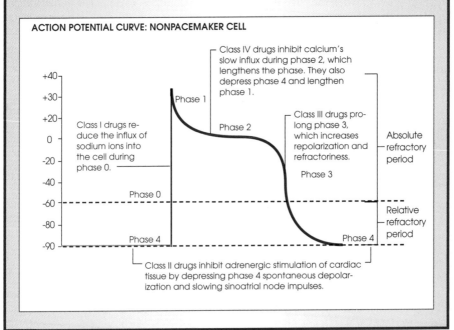

ACTION POTENTIAL CURVE: NONPACEMAKER CELL

Class IV drugs inhibit calcium's slow influx during phase 2, which lengthens the phase. They also depress phase 4 and lengthen phase 1.

Phase 1

Class I drugs reduce the influx of sodium ions into the cell during phase 0.

Phase 2

Class III drugs prolong phase 3, which increases repolarization and refractoriness.

Phase 3

Absolute refractory period

Phase 0

Phase 4

Phase 4

Relative refractory period

Class II drugs inhibit adrenergic stimulation of cardiac tissue by depressing phase 4 spontaneous depolarization and slowing sinoatrial node impulses.

Drug distribution and clearance

When you give an antiarrhythmic drug by infusion, blood levels will initially be high in well-perfused organs, such as the heart, liver, and kidneys. Drug-induced arrhythmias are more likely to occur early in treatment when drug concentrations are higher. Then, as the drug is distributed throughout the rest of the body, drug concentrations in these organs will diminish. With time, as drug concentrations diminish, the risk of toxicity and drug-induced arrhythmias also declines.

Most antiarrhythmic drugs are metabolized in the liver and excreted by the kidneys. As a result, altered blood flow to these organs can affect drug metabolism and clearance and increase the risk of toxicity. Alterations can result from decreased cardiac output, compromised renal function, and concurrent administration of drugs that induce hepatic enzymes.

Proarrhythmic effects

Antiarrhythmic drugs can be *proarrhythmic;* that is, they cause or exacerbate arrhythmias. These arrhythmias may include sustained ventricular tachycardia, ventricular fibrillation, torsades de pointes, and ventricular standstill. The exact mechanisms that trigger proarrhythmias are unknown, but certain factors predispose the patient to them. Major risk factors include fluid and electrolyte imbalances and structural damage to the myocardium, particularly ischemic tissue injury.

When the patient has an electrolyte imbalance, changes in pH and circulating levels of catecholamines may increase the proarrhythmic effect of some antiarrhythmics. In the patient with myocardial ischemia, an antiarrhythmic may not only suppress abnormal rhythms that originate in diseased tissue, but may also depress healthy tissue and can prolong the action potential and delay ventricular repolarization. Arrhythmias result from triggered activity and a reentry mechanism.

When the patient is receiving an antiarrhythmic, be aware of these additional risk factors for proarrhythmias:
- a history of sustained ventricular tachycardia or ventricular fibrillation
- coronary artery disease or significant valvular disease
- severe left ventricular dysfunction
- electrolyte imbalance, particularly hypokalemia or hypomagnesemia
- history of long QT syndrome.

■ *Class I antiarrhythmics*

Class I antiarrhythmics block the influx of sodium into the cell during phase 0 of the action potential. Because phase 0 is also referred to as the *sodium channel* or *fast channel,* these drugs may also be called *sodium channel blockers* or *fast channel blockers.* Class I antiarrhythmics are frequently subdivided into three groups — A, B, and C — according to their interactions with cardiac sodium channels or the drug's effects on the duration of the action potential.

CLASS IA
Class IA antiarrhythmics include disopyramide, procainamide, and quinidine. These drugs lengthen the duration of the action potential, and their interaction with the sodium channels is classified as intermediate. As a result, conductivity is reduced and repolarization is prolonged. These drugs are used to treat supraventricular arrhythmias, such as paroxysmal supraventricular tachycardia, atrial flutter and atrial fibrillation, and ventricular arrhythmias such as premature ventricular contractions. Procainamide is also used to treat recurrent ventricular tachycardia and ventricular fibrillation.

ECG characteristics
Rhythm strip characteristics for a patient taking an antiarrhythmic vary according to the drug's classification. Variations for class IA antiarrhythmics include:

ECG effects of class IA antiarrhythmics

Class IA antiarrhythmics — such as procainamide and quinidine — affect the cardiac cycle in specific ways and lead to specific electrocardiogram (ECG) changes, as shown here. These drugs:
- block sodium influx during phase 0, which depresses the rate of depolarization
- prolong repolarization and the duration of the action potential
- lengthen the refractory period
- decrease contractility.

ECG characteristics of class IA antiarrhythmics:

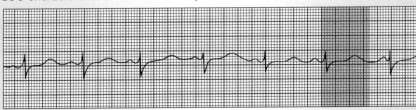

- *QRS complex:* slightly widened
- *QT interval:* prolonged (shaded area)

- QRS complex — slightly widened; increased widening is an early sign of toxicity
- T wave — may be flattened or inverted
- U wave — may be present
- QT interval — prolonged.

RED FLAG Because class IA antiarrhythmics prolong the QT interval, the patient is prone to polymorphic ventricular tachycardia (torsades de pointes). (See *ECG effects of class IA antiarrhythmics.*)

CLASS IB

Class IB antiarrhythmics include lidocaine, mexiletine, tocainide, and phenytoin (rarely used). These agents interact rapidly with sodium channels, slowing phase 0 of the action potential and shortening phase 3. Class IB antiarrhythmics are used in suppressing life-threatening ventricular ectopy, ventricular tachycardia, and ventricular fibrillation.

ECG characteristics

When a patient is taking a class IB antiarrhythmic, check for these ECG changes:
- PR interval — may be prolonged
- QT interval — shortened. (See *ECG effects of class IB antiarrhythmics*, page 186.)

ECG effects of class IB antiarrhythmics

Class IB antiarrhythmics — such as lidocaine and tocainide — may affect the QRS complex, as shown here. They may also:
- block sodium influx during phase 0, which depresses the rate of depolarization
- shorten repolarization and the duration of the action potential
- suppress ventricular automaticity in ischemic tissue.

Electrocardiogram (ECG) characteristics of class IB antiarrhythmics:

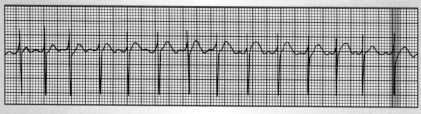

- *PR interval:* may be prolonged
- *QRS complex:* slightly widened (shaded area)

CLASS IC

Class IC antiarrhythmics, including flecainide and propafenone, and moricizine (shares properties of classes IA, IB, and IC) interact slowly with sodium channels. Phase 0 is markedly slowed and conduction is decreased.

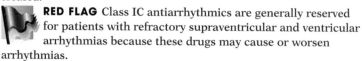 **RED FLAG** Class IC antiarrhythmics are generally reserved for patients with refractory supraventricular and ventricular arrhythmias because these drugs may cause or worsen arrhythmias.

ECG characteristics

When a patient is taking a class IC antiarrhythmic, look for these ECG changes:
- PR interval — prolonged
- QRS complex — widened
- QT interval — prolonged. (See *ECG effects of class IC antiarrhythmics.*)

■ Class II antiarrhythmics

Class II antiarrhythmics include drugs that reduce adrenergic activity in the heart. Beta-adrenergic antagonists, also called *beta blockers,* are class II antiarrhythmics and include such drugs as acebutolol, atenolol, esmolol, metoprolol, and propranolol. Beta-adrenergic antagonists block

ECG effects of class IC antiarrhythmics

Class IC antiarrhythmics — such as flecainide, moricizine, and propafenone — exert particular actions on the cardiac cycle and lead to specific electrocardiogram (ECG) changes, as shown here. These agents block sodium influx during phase 0, which depresses the rate of depolarization. Class IC antiarrhythmics exert no effect on repolarization or the duration of the action potential.

ECG characteristics of class IC antiarrhythmics:

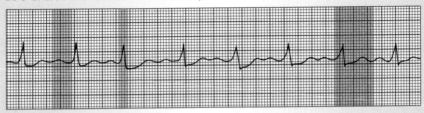

- *PR interval:* prolonged (shaded area, above left)
- *QRS complex:* widened (shaded area, above center)
- *QT interval:* prolonged (shaded area, above right)

beta receptors in the sympathetic nervous system. As a result, phase 4 depolarization is diminished, which leads to depressed automaticity of the sinoatrial node and increased atrial and atrioventricular (AV) node refractory periods.

Class II antiarrhythmics are used to treat supraventricular and ventricular arrhythmias, especially those caused by excess circulating catecholamines. Beta-adrenergic blockers are classified according to their effects. Cardioselective beta-adrenergic blockers block only beta$_1$ receptors, which decrease heart rate, contractility, and conductivity. Noncardioselective beta-adrenergic blockers block beta$_1$ and beta$_2$ receptors and may cause vasoconstriction and bronchospasm because they block beta$_2$ receptors that relax smooth muscle in the bronchi and blood vessels.

 RED FLAG Use class II antiarrhythmics cautiously in patients with pulmonary disease, such as chronic obstructive pulmonary disease because of the risk of bronchospasm.

ECG CHARACTERISTICS

When a patient is taking a class II antiarrhythmic, you may see these ECG changes:
- Rate — atrial and ventricular rates are decreased
- PR interval — slightly prolonged
- QT interval — slightly shortened. (See *ECG effects of class II antiarrhythmics,* page 188.)

ECG effects of class II antiarrhythmics

Class II antiarrhythmics — including such beta-adrenergic blockers as acebutolol, esmolol, and propranolol — exert particular actions on the cardiac cycle and lead to specific electrocardiogram (ECG) changes, as shown here. These drugs:
- depress sinoatrial node automaticity
- shorten the duration of the action potential
- increase the refractory period of atrial and atrioventricular junctional tissues, which slows conduction
- inhibit sympathetic activity.

ECG characteristics of class II antiarrhythmics:

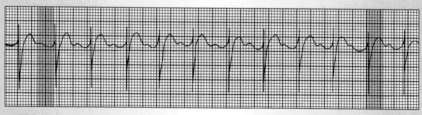

- *PR interval:* slightly prolonged (shaded area, above left)
- *QT interval:* slightly shortened (shaded area, above right)

■ Class III antiarrhythmics

Class III antiarrhythmics prolong the action potential duration, which, in turn, prolongs the effective refractory period. Class III drugs are called *potassium channel blockers* because they block the movement of potassium during phase 3 of the action potential. Drugs in this class include amiodarone, dofetilide, ibutilide, and sotalol (a nonselective beta-adrenergic blocker with mainly class III properties). All class III drugs have proarrhythmic potential. Amiodarone is used to treat rapid atrial arrhythmias and ventricular arrhythmias. Dofetilide is used to treat atrial fibrillation. Ibutilide is used to rapidly convert recent-onset atrial fibrillation or atrial flutter to normal sinus rhythm. Sotalol is used to treat atrial and ventricular arrhythmias.

ECG CHARACTERISTICS

When a patient is taking a class III antiarrhythmic, you may see these ECG changes:
- PR interval — prolonged
- QRS complex — widened
- QT interval — prolonged. (See *ECG effects of class III antiarrhythmics.*)

ECG effects of class III antiarrhythmics

Class III antiarrhythmics — such as amiodarone, ibutilide, and sotalol — affect the cardiac cycle and cause electrocardiogram (ECG) changes, as shown here. These drugs:
- block potassium movement during phase 3
- increase the duration of the action potential
- prolong the effective refractory period.

ECG characteristics of class III antiarrhythmics:

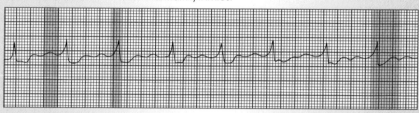

- *PR interval:* prolonged (shaded area, above left)
- *QRS complex:* widened (shaded area, above center)
- *QT interval:* prolonged (shaded area, above right)

■ *Class IV antiarrhythmics*

Class IV antiarrhythmics block the movement of calcium during phase 2 of the action potential. Because phase 2 is also called the *calcium channel* or the *slow channel,* drugs that affect phase 2 are also known as *calcium channel blockers* or *slow channel blockers.* Class IV antiarrhythmics slow conduction and increase the refractory period of calcium-dependent tissues, including the AV node. Drugs in this class include diltiazem and verapamil and are used to treat paroxysmal supraventricular tachycardia, atrial flutter, atrial fibrillation, and multifocal atrial tachycardia.

ECG CHARACTERISTICS

When a patient is taking a class IV antiarrhythmic, check for these ECG changes:
- Rate — atrial and ventricular rates are decreased
- PR interval — prolonged. (See *ECG effects of class IV antiarrhythmics,* page 190.)

ECG effects of class IV antiarrhythmics

Class IV antiarrhythmics — including such calcium channel blockers as diltiazem and verapamil — affect the cardiac cycle in specific ways and may lead to a prolonged PR interval, as shown here. These drugs:

- block calcium movement during phase 2
- prolong the conduction time and increase the refractory period in the atrioventricular node
- decrease contractility.

Electrocardiogram (ECG) characteristics of class IV antiarrhythmics:

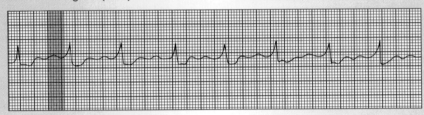

- *PR interval:* prolonged (shaded area)

■ *Digoxin*

Digoxin, the most commonly used cardiac glycoside, works by inhibiting the enzyme adenosine triphosphatase. This enzyme is found in the plasma membrane and acts as a pump to exchange sodium ions for potassium ions. Inhibition of sodium-potassium–activated adenosine triphosphatase results in enhanced movement of calcium from the extracellular space to the intracellular space, thereby strengthening myocardial contractions.

The effects of digoxin on the electrical properties of the heart include direct and autonomic effects. *Direct effects* result in shortening of the action potential, which contributes to the shortening of atrial and ventricular refractoriness. *Autonomic effects* involve the sympathetic and parasympathetic systems. Vagal tone is enhanced, and conduction through the SA and AV nodes is slowed. The drug also exerts an antiarrhythmic effect.

Digoxin is indicated in the treatment of heart failure, paroxysmal supraventricular tachycardia, atrial fibrillation, and atrial flutter.

ECG effects of digoxin

Digoxin affects the cardiac cycle in various ways and may lead to the electrocardiogram (ECG) changes shown here.
ECG characteristics of digoxin:

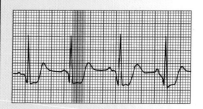

- *ST segment:* gradual sloping, causing ST-segment depression in the opposite direction of the QRS deflection (shaded area)
- *P wave:* may be notched

ECG CHARACTERISTICS

When a patient is taking digoxin, you may see these ECG changes:

- Rate — atrial and ventricular rates are decreased
- PR interval — prolonged
- T wave — decreased
- ST segment — shortened and depressed; sagging (scooping or sloping) of the segment is characteristic
- P wave — may be notched
- QT interval — shortened due to the shortened ST segment. (See *ECG effects of digoxin.*)

RED FLAG Digoxin has a very narrow window of therapeutic effectiveness and, at toxic levels, may cause numerous arrhythmias, including paroxysmal atrial tachycardia with block, AV block, atrial and junctional tachyarrhythmias, and ventricular arrhythmias.

12 *Nonpharmacologic treatment for arrhythmias*

Nonpharmacologic interventions for arrhythmias produce distinctive electrocardiogram (ECG) tracings. These interventions include various types of pacemakers, implantable cardioverter defibrillators, radiofrequency ablation, and ventricular assist devices.

■ *Pacemakers*

A *pacemaker* is an artificial device that electrically stimulates the myocardium to depolarize, initiating mechanical contractions. It works by generating an impulse from a power source and transmitting that impulse to the heart muscle. The impulse flows throughout the heart and causes the heart muscle to depolarize.

A pacemaker may be used when a patient has an arrhythmia, such as certain bradyarrhythmias and tachyarrhythmias, sick sinus syndrome (SSS), or second- and third-degree atrioventricular (AV) block. The device may be used as a temporary measure or a permanent one, depending on the patient's condition. Pacemakers are typically necessary following myocardial infarction or cardiac surgery.

This chapter examines how pacemakers work, ECG characteristics, pacemaker programming, types of pacemakers, pacemaker function assessment, troubleshooting pacemaker problems, interventions, and patient teaching.

PACEMAKER COMPONENTS

A typical pacemaker has three main components: a pulse generator, pacing leads or wires, and one or more electrodes at the distal ends of leadwires. The *pulse generator* contains the pacemaker's power source and circuitry. It creates an electrical impulse that moves through the pacing leads to the electrodes, transmitting that impulse to the heart muscle and causing the heart to depolarize. The lithium battery in a permanent

Understanding pacing leads

Unipolar lead

In a unipolar (one lead) system, electrical current moves from the pulse generator through the leadwire to the negative pole. From there, it stimulates the heart and returns to the pulse generator's metal surface (the positive pole) to complete the circuit.

Bipolar lead

In a bipolar (two lead) system, current flows from the pulse generator through the leadwire to the negative pole at the tip. At that point, it stimulates the heart and then flows back to the positve pole to complete the circuit.

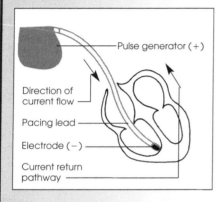

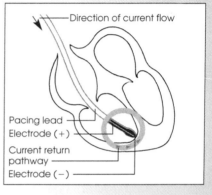

or implanted pacemaker serves as its power source and lasts between 5 and 10 years. A microchip in the device guides heart pacing.

A temporary pacemaker, which isn't implanted, is about the size of a small radio or telemetry box and is powered by alkaline batteries. These units also contain a microchip and are programmed by a touch pad or dials.

An electrical stimulus from the pulse generator moves through wires, or *pacing leads*, to the electrode tips. The leads for a pacemaker, designed to stimulate a single heart chamber, are placed in either the atrium or the ventricle. For dual-chamber, or AV, pacing, the leads are placed in both chambers, usually on the right side of the heart. (See *Understanding pacing leads*.)

The electrodes — one on a unipolar lead or two on a bipolar lead — send information about electrical impulses in the myocardium back to the pulse generator. The pulse generator senses the heart's electrical activity and responds according to how it was programmed.

A *unipolar lead system* is more sensitive to the heart's intrinsic electrical activity than is a bipolar system. A *bipolar system* isn't as easily affected by electrical activity, such as skeletal muscle contraction or magnetic fields, originating outside the heart and the generator. A bipolar system is more difficult to implant, however.

Identifying pacemaker spikes

Pacemaker impulses — the stimuli that travel from the pacemaker to the heart — are visible on an electrocardiogram tracing as spikes. Large or small, pacemaker spikes appear above or below the isoelectric line. This rhythm strip shows an atrial and a ventricular pacemaker spike.

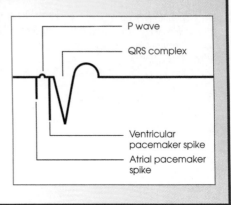

- P wave
- QRS complex
- Ventricular pacemaker spike
- Atrial pacemaker spike

ECG CHARACTERISTICS

The most prominent characteristic of a pacemaker on an ECG is the *pacemaker spike*. (See *Identifying pacemaker spikes*.) It occurs when the pacemaker sends an electrical impulse to the heart muscle. The impulse appears as a vertical line, or spike. The collective group of spikes on an ECG is called *pacemaker artifact*.

Depending on the electrode's position, the spike appears in different locations on the waveform.

- When the pacemaker stimulates the atria, the spike is followed by a P wave and the patient's baseline QRS complex and T wave. This series of waveforms represents successful pacing, or *capture*, of the myocardium. The P wave appears different from the patient's normal P wave.
- When the ventricles are stimulated by a pacemaker, the spike is followed by a QRS complex and a T wave. The QRS complex appears wider than the patient's own QRS complex because of how the pacemaker depolarizes the ventricles.
- When the pacemaker stimulates both the atria and ventricles, the spike is followed by a P wave, then a spike, and then a QRS complex. Be aware that the type of pacemaker used and the patient's condition may affect whether every beat is paced.

■ *Pacemaker programming*

Pacemakers are commonly known by their programmed function and by the number of heart chambers that have a pacing lead. Common programmable functions include rate, mode, output, sensitivity, AV interval, and upper and lower rate limits.

Pacemaker coding system

The capabilities of permanent pacemakers can be described by a five-letter coding system. Typically, only the first three letters are used.

First letter
The first letter identifies which heart chambers are paced:
- V = Ventricle
- A = Atrium
- D = Dual — ventricle and atrium
- 0 = None

Second letter
The second letter signifies the heart chamber where the pacemaker senses intrinsic activity:
- V = Ventricle
- A = Atrium
- D = Dual
- 0 = None

Third letter
The third letter indicates the pacemaker's mode of response to the intrinsic electrical activity it senses in the atrium or ventricle:
- T = Triggers pacing
- I = Inhibits pacing
- D = Dual — can trigger or inhibit depending on the mode and where intrinsic activity occurs
- 0 = None — doesn't change mode in response to sensed activity

Fourth letter
The fourth letter describes the degree of programmability and the presence or absence of an adaptive rate response:
- P = Basic functions programmable
- M = Multiprogrammable parameters
- C = Communicating functions such as telemetry
- R = Rate responsiveness — rate adjusts to fit the patient's metabolic needs and to achieve normal hemodynamic status
- 0 = None

Fifth letter
The fifth letter denotes the pacemaker's response to a tachyarrhythmia:
- P = Pacing ability — pacemaker's rapid burst paces the heart at a rate above its intrinsic rate to override the tachycardia source
- S = Shock — implantable cardioverter-defibrillator identifies ventricular tachycardia and delivers a shock to stop the arrhythmia
- D = Dual ability to shock and pace
- 0 = None

SYNCHRONOUS AND ASYNCHRONOUS PACING
Pacemakers can be classified according to sensitivity. In synchronous, or *demand*, pacing, the pacemaker initiates electrical impulses only when the heart's intrinsic heart rate falls below the preset rate of the pacemaker. In asynchronous, or *fixed*, pacing, the pacemaker constantly initiates electrical impulses at a preset rate without regard to the patient's intrinsic electrical activity or heart rate. This type of pacemaker is rarely used.

PACEMAKER DESCRIPTION CODES
The capabilities of permanent pacemakers are described by a five-letter coding system, though three or four letters are more commonly used. (See *Pacemaker coding system*.)

AAI and VVI pacemakers

AAI and VVI pacemakers are single-chamber pacemakers. The electrode is placed in the atrium for an AAI pacemaker, in the ventricle for a VVI pacemaker. The rhythm strips here show how each pacemaker works.

AAI pacemaker

An AAI pacemaker senses and paces only the atria. As shown in the shaded area below, a P wave follows each atrial spike (atrial depolarization).The QRS complexes reflect the heart's own conduction.

    This pacemaker requires a functioning atrioventricular node and intact conduction system. It may be used in patients who have symptom-producing sinus bradycardia or sick sinus syndrome.

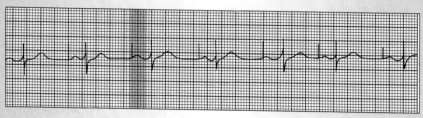

VVI pacemaker

A VVI pacemaker senses and paces the ventricles. When each spike is followed by a QRS complex (depolarization), as shown below, the rhythm is said to reflect 100% capture.

    This pacemaker may be used in patients who have chronic atrial fibrillation with slow ventricular response and those who need infrequent pacing.

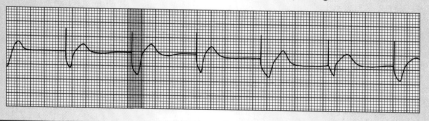

PACING MODES

A pacemaker's *mode* indicates its functions. Several different modes may be used during pacing, and they may not mimic the normal cardiac cycle. A three-letter code, rather than a five-letter code, is typically used to describe pacemaker function. Modes include AAI, VVI, DVI, and DDD. (See *AAI and VVI pacemakers.*)

AAI mode

The AAI, or *atrial demand,* pacemaker is a single-chambered pacemaker that paces and senses the atria. When the pacemaker senses intrinsic atrial activity, it inhibits pacing and resets itself. Only the atria are paced.

DVI pacemakers

A committed DVI pacemaker (also known as an *atrioventricular (AV) sequential pacemaker*) senses ventricular activity and paces the atria and ventricles, firing despite the intrinsic QRS complex.

The rhythm strip here shows the effects of a committed DVI pacemaker. Notice that in two of the complexes (shaded areas), the pacemaker didn't sense the intrinsic QRS complex because the complex occurred during the AV interval, when the pacemaker was already committed to fire.

With a noncommitted DVI pacemaker, spikes wouldn't appear after the QRS complex because the stimulus to pace the ventricles would be inhibited.

Electrocardiogram characteristic of committed DVI pacemaker:

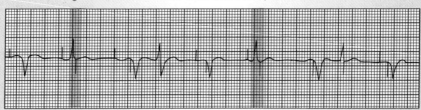

■ Ventricular pacemaker: fires despite the intrinsic QRS complex

Because AAI pacemakers require a functioning AV node and intact conduction system, they aren't used in AV block. An AAI pacemaker may be used in patients with sinus bradycardia, which may occur after cardiac surgery, or with SSS, as long as the AV node and His-Purkinje system aren't diseased.

VVI mode

The VVI, or *ventricular demand,* pacemaker paces and senses the ventricles. When it senses intrinsic ventricular activity, it inhibits pacing.

This single-chambered pacemaker benefits patients with complete heart block and those needing intermittent pacing. Because it doesn't affect atrial activity, it's used for patients who don't need an atrial kick — the extra 15% to 30% of cardiac output that comes from atrial contraction.

If a patient has spontaneous atrial activity, a VVI pacemaker won't synchronize the ventricular activity with it, so tricuspid and mitral insufficiency may develop. Patients who are sedentary may receive this pacemaker, but it won't adjust its rate for patients who are more active.

DVI mode

The DVI, or *AV sequential,* pacemaker paces the atria and ventricles. (See *DVI pacemakers.*) This dual-chambered pacemaker senses only the ventricles' intrinsic activity, inhibiting ventricular pacing.

DDD pacemakers

When evaluating the rhythm strip of a patient with a DDD pacemaker, keep several points in mind.
- If the patient has an adequate intrinsic rhythm, the pacemaker won't fire; it doesn't need to.
- If you see an intrinsic P wave followed by a ventricular pacemaker spike, the pacemaker is tracking the atrial rate and assuring a ventricular response.
- If you see a pacemaker spike before a P wave, followed by an intrinsic ventricular QRS complex, the atrial rate is falling below the lower rate limit, causing the atrial channel to fire. Normal conduction to the ventricles follows.
- If you see a pacemaker spike before a P wave and before the QRS complex, no intrinsic activity is taking place in either the atria or ventricles.

In the rhythm strip shown below, complexes 1, 2, 4, and 7 show the atrial-synchronous mode, set at a rate of 70. The patient has an intrinsic P wave, so the pacemaker only ensures that the ventricles respond. Complexes 3, 5, 8, 10, and 12 are intrinsic ventricular depolarizations. The pacemaker senses them and doesn't fire. In complexes 6, 9, and 11, the pacemaker is pacing the atria and ventricles in sequence. In complex 13, only the atria are paced; the ventricles respond on their own.

Electrocardiogram characteristics of DDD pacemakers:

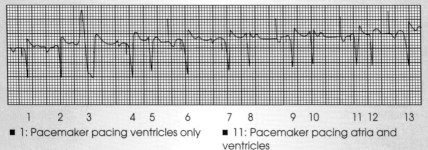

1　　2　　3　　　4　5　　　6　　　7　8　　　9　10　　　11 12　　　13

- 1: Pacemaker pacing ventricles only
- 11: Pacemaker pacing atria and ventricles

Two types of DVI pacemakers may be used, a committed DVI and a noncommitted DVI pacemaker. The *committed DVI pacemaker* doesn't sense intrinsic activity during the AV interval — the time between an atrial and ventricular spike. It generates an impulse even with spontaneous ventricular depolarization. The *noncommitted DVI pacemaker*, on the other hand, is inhibited if a spontaneous depolarization occurs.

The DVI pacemaker helps patients with AV block or SSS who have a diseased His-Purkinje conduction system. It provides the benefits of AV synchrony and atrial kick, thus improving cardiac output. However, it can't vary the atrial rate and isn't helpful in atrial fibrillation because it can't capture the atria. In addition, it may needlessly fire or inhibit its own pacing.

DDD mode

A DDD, or *universal*, pacemaker is used with severe AV block. (See *DDD pacemakers*.) However, because the pacemaker possesses so many capabilities, it may be hard to troubleshoot problems.

Advantages of the DDD pacemaker include its:

- versatility
- programmability
- ability to change modes automatically
- ability to mimic the normal physiologic cardiac cycle, maintaining AV synchrony
- ability to sense and pace the atria and ventricles at the same time according to the intrinsic atrial rate and maximal rate limit.

Unlike other pacemakers, the DDD pacemaker is set with a rate range, rather than a single critical rate. It senses atrial activity and ensures that the ventricles respond to each atrial stimulation, thereby maintaining normal AV synchrony.

The DDD pacemaker fires when the ventricle doesn't respond on its own, and it paces the atria when the atrial rate falls below the lower set rate. In a patient with a high atrial rate, a safety mechanism allows the pacemaker to follow the intrinsic atrial rate only to a preset upper limit. That limit is usually set at about 130 beats/minute and helps to prevent the ventricles from responding to atrial tachycardia or atrial flutter.

■ Types of pacemakers

A pacemaker can be permanent or temporary. Certain pacemakers can pace both the left and right ventricles.

PERMANENT PACEMAKERS

A *permanent pacemaker* is used to treat chronic heart conditions, such as second- and third-degree AV block. It's surgically implanted, usually under local anesthesia. The leads are placed transvenously, positioned in the appropriate chambers, and then anchored to the endocardium. (See *Placing a permanent pacemaker*, page 200.)

The generator is then implanted in a subcutaneous pocket of tissue usually constructed under the patient's clavicle. Most permanent pacemakers are programmed before implantation. The programming sets the conditions under which the pacemaker functions and can be adjusted externally if necessary.

BIVENTRICULAR PACEMAKERS

Biventricular pacing, also referred to as *cardiac resynchronization therapy*, is used to treat patients with moderate and severe heart failure who have left ventricular dyssynchrony. These patients have intraventricular conduction defects, which result in uncoordinated contraction of the

Placing a permanent pacemaker

Implanting a pacemaker is a surgical procedure performed with local anesthesia and moderate sedation. To implant an endocardial pacemaker, the surgeon usually selects a transvenous route and begins lead placement by inserting a catheter percutaneously or by venous cutdown. Then, using fluoroscopic guidance, the surgeon threads the catheter through the vein until the tip reaches the endocardium.

Lead placement
For lead placement in the atrium, the tip must lodge in the right atrium or coronary sinus, as shown here. For placement in the ventricle, it must lodge in the right ventricular apex in one of the interior muscular ridges, or trabeculae.

Implanting the generator
When the lead is in proper position, the surgeon secures the pulse generator in a subcutaneous pocket of tissue just below the patient's clavicle. Changing the generator's battery or microchip circuitry requires only a shallow incision over the site and a quick exchange of components.

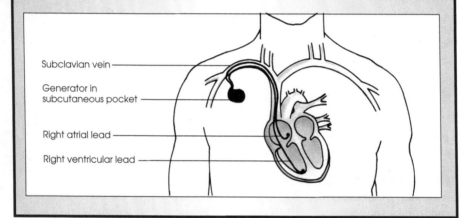

Subclavian vein

Generator in subcutaneous pocket

Right atrial lead

Right ventricular lead

right and left ventricles and a wide QRS complex on an ECG. Left ventricular dyssynchrony has been associated with worsening heart failure and increased morbidity and mortality.

Under normal conditions, the right and left ventricles contract simultaneously to pump blood to the lungs and body, respectively. However, in a patient with heart failure, the damaged ventricles can't pump as forcefully and the amount of blood ejected with each contraction is reduced. If the ventricular conduction pathways are also damaged, electrical impulses reach the ventricles at different times, producing asynchronous contractions (intraventricular conduction defect), which further reduces the amount of blood that the heart pumps, worsening the patient's symptoms.

Biventricular lead placement

The biventricular pacemaker uses three leads: one to pace the right atrium, one to pace the right ventricle, and one to pace the left ventricle. The left ventricular lead is placed in the coronary sinus. Both ventricles are paced at the same time, causing them to contract simultaneously, improving cardiac output

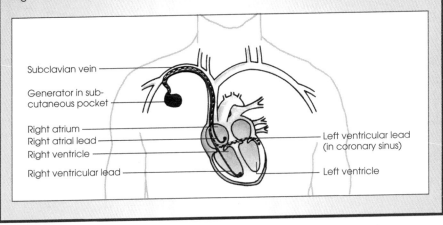

To compensate for this reduced cardiac output, the sympathetic nervous system releases *neurohormones,* such as aldosterone, norepinephrine, and vasopressin, to boost the amount of blood ejected with each contraction. The resultant tachycardia and vasoconstriction increase the heart's demand for oxygen, reduce diastolic filling time, promote sodium and water retention, and increase the pressure that the heart must pump against.

To coordinate ventricular contractions and improve hemodynamic status, biventricular pacemakers use three leads — one in the right atrium and one in each ventricle. Both ventricles are paced at the same time, causing them to contract simultaneously, thereby increasing cardiac output.

Unlike traditional lead placement, the electrode tip for the left ventricle is placed in the coronary sinus to a branch of the inferior cardiac vein. Because this electrode tip isn't anchored in place, lead displacement may occur. (See *Biventricular lead placement.*)

Biventricular pacing produces an immediate improvement in the patient's symptoms and activity tolerance. Moreover, biventricular pacing improves left ventricular remodeling and diastolic function and reduces sympathetic stimulation. As a result, the progression of heart failure is slowed and quality of life is improved in many patients.

Keep in mind, however, that not all patients with heart failure benefit from biventricular pacing. Candidates should have both systolic heart failure and ventricular dyssynchrony along with these characteristics:

■ symptom-producing heart failure despite maximal medical therapy
■ moderate to severe heart failure (New York Heart Association class III or IV)
■ QRS complex greater than 0.13 second
■ left ventricular ejection fraction of 35% or less.

TEMPORARY PACEMAKERS

A *temporary pacemaker* is commonly inserted in an emergency. The patient may show signs of decreased cardiac output, such as hypotension or syncope. The temporary pacemaker supports the patient until the condition resolves.

A temporary pacemaker can also serve as a bridge until a permanent pacemaker is inserted. These pacemakers are used for patients with high-grade heart block, bradycardia, or low cardiac output. Several types of temporary pacemakers are available, including transvenous, epicardial, transcutaneous, and transthoracic.

Transvenous pacemakers

Physicians usually use the transvenous approach — inserting the pacemaker through a vein, such as the subclavian or internal jugular vein — when inserting a temporary pacemaker. The *transvenous pacemaker* is probably the most common and reliable type of temporary pacemaker. It's usually inserted at the bedside or in a fluoroscopy suite. The leadwires are advanced through a catheter into the right ventricle or atrium and then connected to the pulse generator.

Epicardial pacemakers

Epicardial pacemakers are commonly used for patients undergoing cardiac surgery. The tips of the leadwires are attached to the heart's surface and then the wires are brought through the chest wall, below the incision. They're then attached to the pulse generator. The leadwires are usually removed several days after surgery or when the patient no longer requires them.

Transcutaneous pacemakers

Use of a transcutaneous, or *external*, pacemaker has become commonplace in the past several years. In this noninvasive method, there are two placement positions for the electrode pads.
■ Anterior-posterior placement (most common placement):
– Place the anterior (front) electrode pad on the patient's anterior chest wall to the left of the sternum at the fourth and fifth intercostal spaces, halfway between the xiphoid process and left nipple.
– Place the posterior (back) electrode pad on the left side of the back directly behind the anterior pad, just below the scapula to the left of the spine.
■ Anterior-apex placement (alternative placement, if the patient can't tolerate posterior placement):

– Place the anterior (front) electrode pad on the patient's chest wall to the left of the sternum at the fourth and fifth intercostal spaces, midaxillary line.
– Place the posterior (back) electrode pad on the patient's anterior chest wall to the right of the upper sternum below the clavicle at the second or third intercostal space.

An external pulse generator then emits pacing impulses that travel through the patient's skin to the heart muscle. Transcutaneous pacing is built into many defibrillators for use in emergencies. In a transcutaneous pacemaker, the electrodes are built into the same pads used for defibrillation.

Transcutaneous pacing is a quick, noninvasive effective method of pacing heart rhythm and is commonly used in emergencies until a transvenous pacemaker can be inserted. However, some patients may not be able to tolerate the irritating sensations produced from prolonged pacing at the levels needed to pace the heart externally. If the patient is hemodynamically stable, he may require sedation.

Transthoracic pacemakers

A *transthoracic pacemaker* is a type of temporary ventricular pacemaker only used during cardiac emergencies as a last resort. Transthoracic pacing requires insertion of a long needle into the right ventricle, using a subxiphoid approach. A pacing wire is then guided directly into the endocardium.

TEMPORARY PACEMAKER SETTINGS

A temporary pacemaker has several types of settings on the pulse generator. The rate control regulates how many impulses are generated in 1 minute and is measured in pulses per minute (ppm). The rate is usually set at 60 to 80 ppm. (See *Temporary pulse generator,* page 204.) The pacemaker fires if the patient's heart rate falls below the preset rate. The rate may be set higher if the patient has a tachyarrhythmia that's being treated with overdrive pacing.

A pacemaker's energy output is measured in milliamperes, a measurement that represents the stimulation threshold, or how much energy is required to stimulate the cardiac muscle to depolarize. The stimulation threshold is sometimes referred to as *energy required for capture.*

You can also program the pacemaker's sensitivity, measured in millivolts. Most pacemakers allow the patient's heart to function naturally and assist only when necessary. The sensing threshold allows the pacemaker to do this by sensing the heart's normal activity.

INTERVENTIONS

Make sure you're familiar with different types of pacemakers and how they function, so you'll feel more confident in an emergency. When caring for a patient with a pacemaker, follow these guidelines.

Temporary pulse generator

The settings on a temporary pulse generator may be changed in various ways to meet the patient's specific needs. The illustration below shows a single-chamber temporary pulse generator and gives brief descriptions of its various parts.

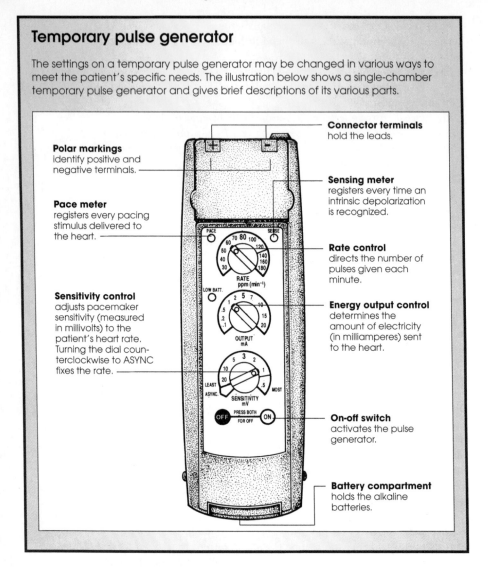

Connector terminals hold the leads.

Polar markings identify positive and negative terminals.

Sensing meter registers every time an intrinsic depolarization is recognized.

Pace meter registers every pacing stimulus delivered to the heart.

Rate control directs the number of pulses given each minute.

Sensitivity control adjusts pacemaker sensitivity (measured in millivolts) to the patient's heart rate. Turning the dial counterclockwise to ASYNC fixes the rate.

Energy output control determines the amount of electricity (in milliamperes) sent to the heart.

On-off switch activates the pulse generator.

Battery compartment holds the alkaline batteries.

For permanent pacemakers

- Use a systematic approach to assess pacemaker function for problems.
  - Identify the mode.
  - Find out what the base rate and upper rate limit (maximum tracking or sensor rate) is.
  - Determine if such features as mode switching or rate response are activated.
  - Find out if the device is a biventricular pacemaker.
  - Determine if the patient is pacemaker-dependent.
  - Identify the patient's signs and symptoms.

- Evaluate all sources of information:
- patient identification card issued by the pacemaker manufacturer
- patient history
- patient or family knowledge of device function
- physician notes, printouts from programmer if available
- ECG observation.
- Review the patient's 12-lead ECG to evaluate pacemaker function. If unavailable, examine lead V_1 or modified chest lead$_1$ (MCL_1) instead.
- Select a monitoring lead that clearly shows the pacemaker spikes and compare at least two leads to verify what you observe.
- Remember: Visibility of spikes depends on pacing polarity and type of lead.
- Measure the rate and interpret the paced rhythm.
- Compare the morphology of paced and intrinsic complexes (traditional right ventricular pacing should produce a morphology similar to left bundle-branch block pattern).
- Differentiate between ventricular ectopy and paced activity.
- Look for information that tells you which chamber is paced and information about the pacemaker's sensing function.
- Monitor the patient's vital signs.
- Look for evidence of problems:
- decreased cardiac output (hypotension, chest pain, dyspnea, syncope)
- infection
- pneumothorax
- abnormal electrical stimulation occurring in synchrony with the pacemaker
- pectoral muscle twitching
- hiccups (stimulation of diaphragm)
- cardiac tamponade.
- Know that placing a magnet over the pulse generator makes the pacemaker temporarily revert to an asynchronous mode (safety mode) at a preset rate. (See *Assessing pacemaker function,* page 206.)

For biventricular pacemakers
Provide the same basic care to the patient with a biventricular pacemaker that you would give a patient with a standard permanent pacemaker. Specific care includes these guidelines:
- Because of the position of the left ventricular lead, watch for stimulation of the diaphragm and left chest wall. Notify the physician if this occurs because the left ventricular lead may need repositioning.
- Observe the ECG for pacemaker spikes. Although both ventricles are paced, only one pacemaker spike is seen.
- Measure the duration of the QRS complex. Typically, you'll observe a narrowing of the QRS complex. A widened QRS complex may indicate that the left ventricular lead is no longer positioned properly.

Assessing pacemaker function

When you apply a magnet to a patient's pacemaker, the device reverts to a predefined (asynchronous) response mode that allows you to assess various aspects of pacemaker function. Specifically, you can:

■ determine which chambers are being paced
■ assess capture
■ provide emergency pacing if the device malfunctions
■ ensure pacing despite electromagnetic interference
■ assess battery life by checking the magnet rate — a predetermined rate that indicates the need for battery replacement.

Keep in mind, however, that you must know which implanted device the patient has before you consider using a magnet on it. The patient might have an implantable cardioverter-defibrilla-tor (ICD), which is only rarely an appropriate target for magnet application.

What's more, because pacemaker and ICDs are similar in generator size and implant location, it's not as easy to differentiate between the two. In addition, a single device may perform multiple functions.

In general, you shouldn't apply a magnet to an ICD or a pacemaker-ICD combination. Applying a magnet to an ICD can cause an unexpected response because various responses can be programmed or determined by the manufacturer. When directed, applying a magnet to an ICD usually suspends therapies for ventricular tachycardia and fibrillation while leaving bradycardia pacing active, which may be helpful in patients who receive multiple, inappropriate shocks. Some models may beep when exposed to a magnetic field.

For temporary pacemakers

■ Check stimulation and sensing thresholds daily because they increase over time.

■ Assess the patient and pacemaker regularly to check for possible problems:
 – failure to capture
 – failure to pace
 – undersensing
 – oversensing.

■ Turn or reposition the patient carefully to prevent dislodgment of the leadwire.

■ Follow recommended electrical safety precautions.

■ Avoid microshocks to the patient by making sure that the bed and all electrical equipment is grounded properly and that all pacing wires and connections to temporary wires are insulated with moisture-proof material (such as a disposable glove).

■ Obtain a chest X-ray and assist the physician with repositioning the leadwire if required.

 RED FLAG All invasive temporary pacing has the potential to deliver a shock directly to the heart along the pacing wire, resulting in ventricular tachycardia or fibrillation.

- Defibrillation and cardioversion (up to 360 joules) don't usually require that the pulse generator be disconnected.
- Look for evidence of problems:
- decreased cardiac output (hypotension, chest pain, dyspnea, syncope)
- infection
- pneumothorax
- abnormal electrical stimulation occurring in synchrony with the pacemaker
- pectoral muscle twitching
- hiccups (stimulation of diaphragm)
- signs of a perforated ventricle and the resultant cardiac tamponade. Signs and symptoms include persistent hiccups, tachycardia, distant heart sounds, pulsus paradoxus (indicated by a drop in the strength of a pulse during inspiration), hypotension with narrowed pulse pressure, cyanosis, distended jugular veins, decreased urine output, restlessness, and complaints of fullness in the chest. Notify the physician immediately if you note any of these signs and symptoms.
- If there's no output (pacing is required but the pacemaker fails to stimulate the heart), take these steps:
- Verify that the pacemaker is on.
- Check the output settings.
- Change the pulse generator battery.
- Change the pulse generator.
- Check for disconnection or dislodgment of the pacing wire.

EVALUATING PACEMAKER FUNCTION

After a pacemaker has been implanted, its function should be assessed. First, determine the pacemaker's mode and settings. If the patient had a permanent pacemaker implanted before admission, ask whether the wallet card from the manufacturer notes the mode and settings.

If the pacemaker was recently implanted, check the patient's medical record for information about the pacemaker settings because this precaution will help prevent misinterpretation of the ECG tracing. For instance, if the tracing has ventricular spikes but no atrial pacing spikes, you might assume that it's a VVI pacemaker when it could be a DVI pacemaker that has lost its atrial output.

Next, review the patient's 12-lead ECG. If it isn't available, examine lead V_1 or MCL_1 instead.

Select a monitoring lead that clearly shows the pacemaker spikes. Make sure the lead you select doesn't cause the cardiac monitor to misinterpret a spike for a QRS complex and double-count the heart rate. This misinterpretation may cause the alarm to sound, falsely signaling a high heart rate.

When looking at an ECG tracing for a patient with a pacemaker, consider the pacemaker mode, and then interpret the paced rhythm. Does it correlate with what you know about the pacemaker?

Look for information that tells you which chamber is paced. Is there capture? Is there a P wave or QRS complex after each atrial or ventricular spike? Or do the P waves and QRS complexes stem from intrinsic electrical activity?

Look for information about the pacemaker's sensing ability. If intrinsic atrial or ventricular activity is present, what's the pacemaker's response?

Look at the rate. What's the pacing rate per minute? Is it appropriate given the pacemaker settings? Although you can determine the rate quickly by counting the number of complexes in a 6-second ECG strip, a more accurate method is to count the number of small boxes between complexes and divide this number into 1,500.

Knowing your patient's medical history and whether a pacemaker has been implanted will also help you to determine whether your patient is experiencing ventricular ectopy or paced activity on the ECG. (See *Distinguishing intermittent ventricular pacing from PVCs.*)

PATIENT TEACHING

Following pacemaker insertion, explain to the patient why a pacemaker is needed, how it works, and what can be expected from it. Be sure to cover these points with the patient and his family.

For permanent pacemakers
- Provide information to the patient about:
  - pacemaker's function
  - related anatomy and physiology
  - patient's indication for pacemaker
  - postoperative care and routines.
- Provide discharge instructions, which usually include these topics:
  - incision care
  - signs of pocket complications (hematoma, infection, bleeding)
  - avoidance of heavy lifting or vigorous activity for 2 to 4 weeks
  - limited arm movement on side of pacemaker
  - medical follow-up
  - transtelephonic monitoring follow-up if indicated
  - identification card to be carried
  - procedure for taking pulse.
- Explain signs and symptoms to report to physician:
  - light-headedness, syncope, fatigue, palpitations, muscle stimulation, hiccups
  - slow (below the base rate) or unusually fast heart rate.
- Because today's pacemakers are well shielded from environmental interactions, explain that the patient can safely use:
  - most common household appliances, including microwaves
  - cellular phones (on the opposite side of pacemaker)

LOOK-ALIKES

Distinguishing intermittent ventricular pacing from PVCs

Knowing whether your patient has an artificial pacemaker will help you avoid mistaking a ventricular paced beat for a premature ventricular contraction (PVC). If your facility uses a monitoring system that eliminates artifact, make sure the monitor is set up correctly for a patient with a pacemaker. Otherwise, the pacemaker spikes may be eliminated as well.

If your patient has intermittent ventricular pacing, the paced ventricular complex will have a pacemaker spike preceding it as shown in the shaded area of the top electrocardiogram (ECG) strip. You may need to look in different leads for a bipolar pacemaker spike because it's small and may be difficult to see. What's more, the paced ventricular complex of a properly functioning pacemaker won't occur early or prematurely, it will occur only when the patient's own ventricular rate falls below the rate set for the pacemaker.

If your patient is having PVCs, they'll occur prematurely and won't have pacemaker spikes preceding them. Examples are shown in the shaded areas of the bottom ECG strip.

INTERMITTENT VENTRICULAR PACING

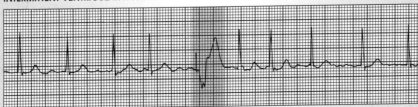

PVCs

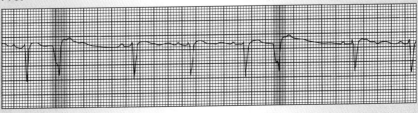

– spark-ignited combustion engines (leaf blower, lawnmower, automobile)
– office equipment (computer, copier, fax machine)
– light shop equipment.
■ Caution the patient to avoid close or prolonged exposure to potential sources of electromagnetic interference. (See *Understanding EMI*, page 210.)
■ Remind the patient about travel-related issues:

Understanding EMI

Electromagnetic interference (EMI) can wreak havoc in patients who have a pacemaker or an implantable cardioverter-defibrillator (ICD). For those with a pacemaker, EMI may inhibit pacing, cause asynchronous or unnecessary pacing, or mimic intrinsic cardiac activity. For those with an ICD, EMI may mimic ventricular fibrillation, or it may prevent detection of a problem that needs treatment.

If your patient has a pacemaker or an ICD, review common sources of EMI and urge him to avoid them. EMIs may include:

- strong electromagnetic fields
- large generators and transformers
- arc and resistance welders
- large magnets
- motorized radiofrequency equipment.

EMI may present a risk in health care facility settings as well. Make sure your patient knows to notify all health care providers about the implanted device so the provider can evaluate the risk of such therapies as:

- magnetic resonance imaging (usually contraindicated)
- radiation therapy (excluding diagnostic X-rays, such as mammograms, which typically are safe)
- diathermy
- electrocautery
- transcutaneous electrical nerve stimulation.

– Metal detectors don't disturb pacemaker function but may detect the device.

– Handheld scanning tools shouldn't be used over the pacemaker or near it.

– An identification card may be needed to show security personnel.

For biventricular pacemakers

Provide the same basic teaching that you would give to the patient receiving a permanent pacemaker. Additionally, when a patient has a biventricular pacemaker, be sure to cover these points:

- Explain to the patient and his family why a biventricular pacemaker is needed, how it works, and what they can expect.
- Tell the patient and his family that it's sometimes difficult to place the left ventricular lead and that the procedure can take 3 hours or more.
- Stress the importance of calling the physician immediately if the patient develops chest pain, shortness of breath, swelling of the hands or feet, or a weight gain of 3 lb (1.4 kg) in 24 hours or 5 lb (2.3 kg) in 48 to 72 hours.

For temporary pacemakers

- Provide information to the patient about the temporary pacemaker's function, related anatomy and physiology, the need for the pacemaker, and potential need for a permanent pacemaker.
- Explain postprocedure care and pain management.
- Advise the patient not to get out of bed without assistance.
- Instruct the patient not to manipulate the pacemaker wires or pulse generator.

■ Explain symptoms to report to the nurse, such as light-headedness, syncope, palpitations, muscle stimulation, or hiccups.
■ Advise the patient to limit arm movement on the same side of the pacemaker.

TROUBLESHOOTING PACEMAKER PROBLEMS

A malfunctioning pacemaker can lead to arrhythmias, hypotension, syncope, and other signs and symptoms of decreased cardiac output. (See *Recognizing a malfunctioning pacemaker*, pages 212 and 213.) Common problems with pacemakers that can lead to low cardiac output and loss of AV synchrony include:
■ failure to capture
■ failure to pace
■ undersensing
■ oversensing.

Failure to capture

Failure to capture appears on an ECG as a pacemaker spike without the appropriate atrial or ventricular response — a spike without a complex. Think of failure to capture as the pacemaker's inability to stimulate the chamber.

Causes of failure to capture include acidosis, electrolyte imbalances, fibrosis, incorrect leadwire position, a low mA or output setting, depletion of the battery, a broken or cracked leadwire, or perforation of the leadwire through the myocardium.

Failure to pace

Failure to pace is indicated by no pacemaker activity on an ECG when pacemaker activity is appropriately expected. This problem may be caused by battery or circuit failure, cracked or broken leads, or interference between atrial and ventricular sensing in a dual-chambered pacemaker. Failure to pace can lead to asystole.

Undersensing

Undersensing is indicated by a pacemaker spike when intrinsic cardiac activity is present. In asynchronous pacemakers that have codes, such as VOO or DOO, undersensing is a programming limitation.

When undersensing occurs in synchronous pacemakers, pacing spikes occur on the ECG where they shouldn't. Although they may appear in any part of the cardiac cycle, the spikes are especially dangerous if they fall on the T wave, where they can cause ventricular tachycardia or ventricular fibrillation.

In synchronous pacemakers, undersensing may be caused by electrolyte imbalances, disconnection or dislodgment of a lead, improper lead placement, increased sensing threshold from edema or fibrosis at the electrode tip, drug interactions, or a depleted pacemaker battery.

Recognizing a malfunctioning pacemaker

Occasionally, pacemakers fail to function properly. When this happens, you'll need to take immediate action to correct the problem. The rhythm strips below show examples of problems that can occur with a temporary or permanent pacemaker.

Failure to capture

- Electrocardiogram (ECG) shows a pacemaker spike without the appropriate atrial or ventricular response (spike without a complex), as shown at right.
- Patient may be asymptomatic or have signs of decreased cardiac output.
- Pacemaker can't stimulate the chamber.
- Problem may be caused by increased pacing thresholds related to certain situations:
  - Metabolic or electrolyte imbalance
  - Antiarrhythmic use
  - Fibrosis or edema at electrode tip

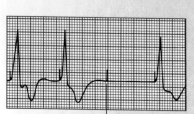

There's a pacemaker spike but no response from the heart.

- Problem may be caused by lead malfunction:
  - Dislodged lead
  - Broken or damaged lead
  - Perforation of myocardium by lead
  - Loose connection between lead and pulse generator
- Related interventions may solve the problem:
  - Treat metabolic disturbance.
  - Replace damaged lead.
  - Change pulse generator battery.
  - Slowly increase output setting on the temporary pacemaker until capture occurs.
  - Determine electrode placement with a chest X-ray if needed.

Failure to pace

- ECG shows no pacemaker activity when pacemaker activity should be evident, as shown at right.
- Magnet application yields no response. (It should cause asynchronous pacing.)
- Problem has several common causes, including:
  - depleted battery
  - circuit failure
  - lead malfunction

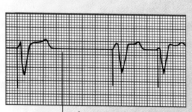

A pacemaker spike should appear here but doesn't.

  - inappropriate programming of sensing function
  - electromagnetic interference.
- Failure to pace can lead to asystole or a severe decrease in cardiac output in the patient who is pacemaker dependent.
- If you think a pacemaker is failing to pace, a temporary pacemaker (transcutaneous or transvenous) should be used to prevent asystole.

Recognizing a malfunctioning pacemaker *(continued)*

- Related interventions may solve the problem:
  - Replace pulse generator battery.
  - Replace pulse generator unit.
  - Adjust sensitivity setting.
  - Remove source of electromagnetic interference.

Failure to sense intrinsic beats (undersensing)

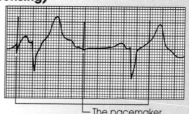

- ECG may show pacing spikes anywhere in the cycle, as shown at right.
- A pacemaker spike may appear where intrinsic cardiac activity is present.
- Patient may report feeling palpitations or skipped beats.
- Spikes are especially dangerous if they fall on the T wave because ventricular tachycardia or fibrillation may result.

└─ The pacemaker fires anywhere in the cycle.

- Problem has several common causes, including:
  - battery failure
  - fracture of pacing leadwire
  - displacement of electrode tip
  - "cross-talk" between atrial and ventricular channels
  - electromagnetic interference mistaken for intrinsic signals.
- Related interventions may solve the problem:
  - Replace the pulse generator battery.
  - Replace the leadwires.
  - Adjust the sensitivity setting.

Oversensing

Oversensing occurs if the pacemaker is too sensitive and it can misinterpret muscle movements or other events in the cardiac cycle as intrinsic cardiac electrical activity. Pacing won't occur when it's needed, and the heart rate and AV synchrony won't be maintained.

■ Implantable cardioverter-defibrillator

An *implantable cardioverter-defibrillator* (ICD) is an electronic device implanted in the patient's body to provide continuous monitoring of the heart for bradycardia, ventricular tachycardia, and ventricular fibrillation. The device then administers either shocks or paced beats to treat the dangerous arrhythmia. In general, ICDs are indicated for patients for whom drug therapy, surgery, or catheter ablation has failed to prevent the arrhythmia.

Types of ICD therapies

An implantable cardioverter-defibrillator (ICD) can deliver a range of therapies depending on the type of device, how the device is programmed, and the arrhythmia it detects. Therapies include antitachycardia pacing, cardioversion, defibrillation, and bradycardia pacing.

Therapy	Description
ANTITACHYCARDIA PACING	A series of small, rapid electrical pacing pulses are used to interrupt atrial fibrillation (AF) or ventricular tachycardia (VT) and return the heart to its normal rhythm. Antitachycardia pacing isn't appropriate for all patients and begins only after appropriate electrophysiology studies.
CARDIOVERSION	A low- or high-energy shock (up to 35 joules) is timed to the R wave to terminate VT and return the heart to its normal rhythm.
DEFIBRILLATION	A high-energy shock (up to 35 joules) is given to the heart to terminate ventricular fibrillation and return the heart to its normal rhythm.
BRADYCARDIA PACING	Electrical pacing pulses are used when natural electrical signals are too slow. ICDs can sense and pace one chamber (VVI pacing) of the heart at a preset rate, both chambers (DDD pacing), or function as a biventricular pacemaker.

Today's advanced devices can detect a wide range of arrhythmias and automatically respond with the appropriate therapy, such as bradycardia pacing (both single- and dual-chamber), antitachycardia pacing, cardioversion, and defibrillation. ICDs that provide therapy for atrial arrhythmias, such as atrial fibrillation, are also available. (See *Types of ICD therapies*.)

The procedure for ICD insertion is similar to that of a permanent pacemaker and may take place in a cardiac catheterization laboratory. Occasionally, a patient who requires other surgery, such as coronary artery bypass grafting, may have the device implanted in the operating room. (See *Reviewing ICDs*.)

An ICD consists of a programmable pulse generator and one or more leadwires. The pulse generator is a small battery-powered computer that monitors the heart's electrical signals and delivers electrical therapy when it identifies an abnormal rhythm. The leads are insulated wires that carry the heart signal to the pulse generator and deliver the electrical energy from the pulse generator to the heart.

An ICD also stores information about the heart's activity before, during, and after an arrhythmia, along with tracking which treatment was delivered and the treatment's outcome. Many devices also store electrograms (electrical tracings similar to ECGs). With an interrogation device,

Reviewing ICDs

Today's implantable cardioverter-defibrillators (ICDs) are easier to implant and more effective than ever. For most patients, the leads can be threaded through the cephalic vein and positioned in the heart and superior vena cava. The pulse generator is inserted under the skin through a small incision. In some cases, a high-voltage subcutaneous patch electrode is placed inside the superior periaxial area to reduce the amount of energy needed for defibrillation.

Programming features have evolved greatly and now allow tiered therapy, antitachycardia pacing, low-energy cardioversion, antibradycardia pacing, data storage, and diagnostic algorithms. In addition, some ICDs allow the magnet mode (in which placing a magnet over the generator suppresses ICD programming) to be turned on or off. With the magnet mode turned off, a magnet won't affect ICD function. In some devices, a magnet temporarily suspends detection and tachycardia therapy, while leaving antibradycardia pacing intact.

Originally, the only patients chosen to receive ICDs were those who survived sudden cardiac death and those who sustained ventricular tachycardia and syncope unresponsive to antiarrhythmics. However, recent reports have revealed a survival rate 40% to 60% higher among at-risk patients with ICDs than among those who received conventional therapies. Consequently, ICDs are now recommended or being investigated for:
- ventricular fibrillation without structural heart disease or triggering factors
- syncope of an undetermined cause
- unsuccessful antiarrhythmic therapy
- patients with risk factors for ventricular arrhythmias
- patients with extensive anterior wall myocardial infarction (MI) who can't take thrombolytic agents
- patients with previous MI and unexplained recurrent syncope
- children with congenital long QT-interval syndrome
- patients who are waiting for heart transplantations.

a physician can retrieve this information to evaluate ICD function and battery status and to adjust ICD system settings.

INTERVENTIONS

When caring for a patient with an ICD, it's important to know how the device is programmed. This information is available through a status report that can be obtained and printed by a physician or specially trained technician. This retrieval involves placing a specialized piece of equipment over the implanted pulse generator to retrieve pacing function. If the patient experiences an arrhythmia or the ICD delivers a therapy, the program information recorded helps to evaluate the functioning of the device.

Program information includes:
- type and model of ICD
- status of the device (on or off)
- detection rates
- therapies that will be delivered: pacing, antitachycardia pacing, cardioversion, and defibrillation.

If your patient experiences an arrhythmia:
■ Assess the patient for signs and symptoms related to decreased cardiac output.
■ Record the patient's ECG rhythm.
■ Evaluate the appropriateness of any delivered ICD therapy.
■ If the patient experiences cardiac arrest, initiate cardiopulmonary resuscitation (CPR) and advanced cardiac life support.
■ If the patient needs external defibrillation, position the paddles as far from the device as possible or use the anteroposterior paddle position.

PATIENT TEACHING
■ Explain to the patient and his family why an ICD is needed, how it works, potential complications, and what they can expect. Make sure they also understand ICD terminology.
■ Discuss signs and symptoms to report to the physician immediately.
■ Advise the patient to wear a medical identification bracelet indicating ICD placement.
■ Educate family members in emergency techniques (such as dialing 911 and performing CPR) in case the device fails.
■ Explain that electrical or electronic devices may cause disruption of the device.
■ Advise the patient to avoid placing excessive pressure over the insertion site or moving or jerking the area until the postoperative visit.
■ Tell the patient to follow normal routines as allowed by the physician and to increase exercise as tolerated. After the first 24 hours, show the patient how to perform passive range-of-motion exercises and progress as tolerated.
■ Remind the patient to carry information regarding his ICD at all times and to inform airline clerks when he travels as well as individuals performing diagnostic studies (such as computed tomography scans and magnetic resonance imaging).
■ Stress the importance of follow-up care and checkups.

■ Radiofrequency ablation

Radiofrequency ablation is an invasive procedure that may be used to treat arrhythmias in patients who haven't responded to antiarrhythmics or cardioversion or can't tolerate antiarrhythmics. In this procedure, a burst of radiofrequency energy is delivered through a catheter to the heart tissue to destroy the arrhythmia's focus or block the conduction pathway.

Radiofrequency ablation is effective in treating patients with atrial fibrillation and flutter, ventricular tachycardia, AV nodal reentry tachycardia, and Wolff-Parkinson-White (WPW) syndrome.

PROCEDURE

The patient first undergoes electrophysiology studies to identify and map the specific area of the heart that's causing the arrhythmia. The ablation catheters are inserted into a vein, usually the femoral vein, and advanced to the heart where short bursts of radiofrequency waves destroy a small targeted area of heart tissue. The destroyed tissue can no longer conduct electrical impulses. Other types of energy may also be used, such as microwave, sonar, or cryo (freezing). In some patients, the tissue inside the pulmonary vein is responsible for the arrhythmia. Targeted radiofrequency ablation is used to block these abnormal impulses. (See *Using radiofrequency ablation,* page 218.)

If a rapid arrhythmia that originates above the AV node (such as atrial fibrillation) isn't terminated by targeted ablation, AV nodal ablation may be used to block electrical impulses from being conducted to the ventricles. After ablation of the AV node, the patient may need a pacemaker because impulses can no longer be conducted from the atria to the ventricles. If the atria continue to beat irregularly, anticoagulation therapy will also be needed to reduce the risk of stroke.

If the patient has WPW syndrome, electrophysiology studies can locate the accessory pathway and ablation can destroy it. When reentry is the cause of the arrhythmia, such as AV nodal reentry tachycardia, ablation can destroy the pathway without affecting the AV node.

INTERVENTIONS

When caring for a patient after radiofrequency ablation, follow these guidelines:

- Provide continuous cardiac monitoring, assessing for arrhythmias and ischemic changes.
- Place the patient on bed rest for 8 hours, or as ordered, and keep the affected extremity straight. Maintain the head of the bed between 15 and 30 degrees.
- Assess the patient's vital signs every 15 minutes for the first hour, then every 30 minutes for 4 hours, unless the patient's condition warrants more frequent checking.
- Assess peripheral pulses distal to the catheter insertion site as well as the color, sensation, temperature, and capillary refill of the affected extremity.
- Check the catheter insertion site for bleeding and hematoma formation.
- Monitor the patient for complications, such as hemorrhage, stroke, perforation of the heart, arrhythmias, phrenic nerve damage, pericarditis, pulmonary vein stenosis or thrombosis, and sudden death.

PATIENT TEACHING

When a patient undergoes radiofrequency ablation, be sure to cover these points:

Using radiofrequency ablation

In radiofrequency ablation, special catheters are inserted in a vein and advanced to the heart. After the arrhythmia's source is identified, radiofrequency energy is used to destroy the source of the abnormal electrical impulses or abnormal conduction pathway.

AV nodal ablation

If a rapid arrhythmia originates above the atrioventricular (AV) node, the AV node may be destroyed to block impulses from reaching the ventricles. The radiofrequency ablation catheter is directed to the AV node (A). Radiofrequency energy is used to destroy the AV node (B).

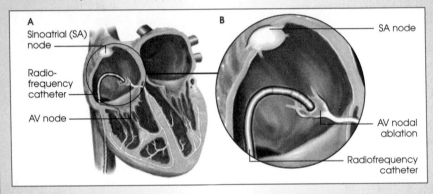

Pulmonary vein ablation

If the pulmonary vein is the source of the arrhythmia, radiofrequency energy is used to destroy the tissue at the base of the pulmonary vein. The radiofrequency catheter is directed to the base of the pulmonary vein (A). Radiofrequency energy is used to destroy the tissue at the base of the pulmonary vein (B).

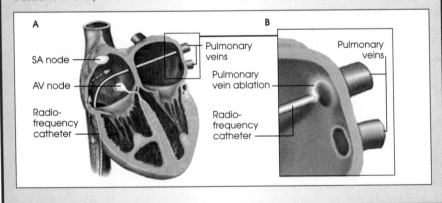

- Discuss with the patient and his family why radiofrequency ablation is needed, how it works, and what they can expect.
- Explain to the patient and his family that the procedure can be lengthy, up to 6 hours if electrophysiology studies are being done first.

- Explain that the patient may be hospitalized for 24 to 48 hours to monitor his heart rhythm.
- Provide pacemaker teaching if the patient had a pacemaker inserted.

■ *Ventricular assist devices*

Ventricular assist devices (VADs) are designed to decrease the heart's workload and increase cardiac output in patients with ventricular failure. Left ventricular, right ventricular, and biventricular VADs are available. (See *How VAD helps a failing heart,* page 220.)

Because a VAD supports the heart's pumping function rather than altering electrical function, it doesn't affect the heart's electrical activity. As a result, you probably won't see ECG changes caused by the VAD.

VADs may be indicated for patients who can't be weaned from cardiopulmonary bypass or intra-aortic balloon pump as well as for patients who are awaiting heart transplantation.

In a surgical procedure, blood is diverted from a ventricle to an artificial pump, which maintains systemic perfusion. VADs are commonly used as a bridge to maintain perfusion until a heart transplantation procedure can be performed.

A VAD is used to provide systemic or pulmonary support, or both:
- A right VAD provides pulmonary support by diverting blood from the failing right ventricle to the VAD, which then pumps the blood to the pulmonary circulation by way of the VAD connection to the pulmonary artery.
- With a left VAD, blood flows from the left ventricle to the VAD, which then pumps blood back to the body by way of the VAD connection to the aorta.
- When biventricular support is needed, both may be used.

INTERVENTIONS
When caring for a patient with a VAD, follow these guidelines:

Patient preparation
- Prepare the patient and his family for insertion, reinforcing explanations about the device, its purpose, and what to expect after insertion.
- Make sure that informed consent is obtained.
- Continue close patient monitoring, including continuous ECG monitoring, pulmonary artery and hemodynamic status monitoring, and intake and output monitoring.

Monitoring and aftercare
- Assess the patient's cardiovascular status, monitor blood pressure and hemodynamic parameters, including cardiac output and cardiac index, ECG, and peripheral pulses.
- Inspect the incision and dressing at least every hour initially and then every 2 to 4 hours as indicated by the patient's condition.

How VAD helps a failing heart

A ventricular assist device (VAD), which is commonly called a *bridge to transplant*, is a mechanical pump that relieves the ventricle's workload as the heart heals or until a donor heart is located.

Implantable
The typical VAD is implanted in the upper abdominal wall. An inflow cannula drains blood from the left ventricle into a pump, which then pushes the blood into the aorta through the outflow cannula.

Pump options
VADs are available as continuous-flow or pulsatile pumps. A *continuous-flow pump* fills continuously and returns blood to the aorta at a constant rate. A *pulsatile pump* may work in one of two ways: It may fill during systole and pump blood into the aorta during diastole, or it may pump irrespective of the patient's cardiac cycle.

Many types of VAD systems are available. The illustration below shows a VAD (from Baxter Novacor) implanted in the left abdominal wall and connected to an external controller by a percutaneous lead. The patient also has a reserve power pack. The monitor is a backup power source that can run on electricity.

Potential complications
Despite the use of anticoagulants, the VAD may cause thrombi formation, leading to pulmonary embolism, transient ischemic attack, or stroke. Other complications may include heart failure, bleeding, cardiac tamponade, infection, sepsis, or device failure.

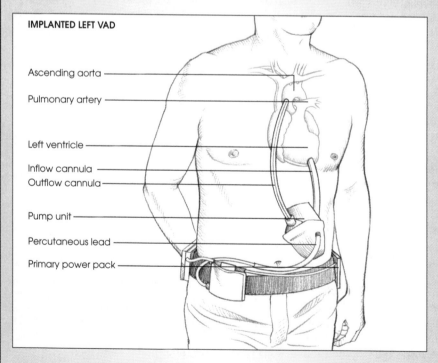

IMPLANTED LEFT VAD

Ascending aorta

Pulmonary artery

Left ventricle

Inflow cannula
Outflow cannula

Pump unit

Percutaneous lead

Primary power pack

■ Monitor urine output hourly, and maintain I.V. fluid therapy as ordered. Watch for signs of fluid overload or decreasing urine output.

■ Assess chest tube drainage and function frequently. Notify the physician if drainage is greater than 150 ml over 2 hours. Auscultate lungs for evidence of abnormal breath sounds or adventitious sounds. Evaluate oxygen saturation or mixed venous oxygen saturation levels, and administer oxygen as needed and ordered.

■ Obtain hemoglobin levels, hematocrit, and coagulation studies as ordered. Administer blood component therapy as indicated and ordered.

■ Assess for signs and symptoms of bleeding.

■ Administer antibiotics prophylactically as ordered to prevent infection.

PATIENT TEACHING

Before discharge after the insertion of a VAD, instruct the patient to:

■ immediately report redness, swelling, or drainage at the incision site; chest pain; or fever

■ immediately notify the physician if signs or symptoms of heart failure (weight gain, dyspnea, or edema) develop

■ follow the prescribed medication regimen and report adverse effects

■ follow his prescribed diet, especially sodium and fat restrictions

■ maintain a balance between activity and rest

■ follow his exercise or rehabilitation program (if prescribed)

■ comply with the laboratory schedule for monitoring International Normalized Ratio if the patient is receiving warfarin (Coumadin).

Part V
Reviewing
rhythm strips

13 *Practice strips*

■ *Sharpening interpretation skills*

Use these sample rhythm strips as a practical way to sharpen your electrocardiogram (ECG) interpretation skills. Record the rhythm, rates, and waveform characteristics in the blank spaces provided, and then compare your findings with the answers beginning on page 234.

1.

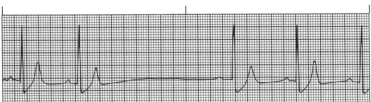

Atrial rhythm: _____
Ventricular rhythm: _____
Atrial rate: _____
Ventricular rate: _____
P wave: _____
PR interval: _____
QRS complex: _____
QT interval: _____
Other: _____
Interpretation: _____

2.

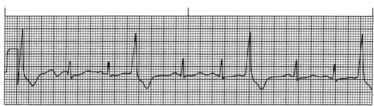

Atrial rhythm: _____

Ventricular rhythm: _____

Atrial rate: _____

Ventricular rate: _____

P wave: _____

PR interval: _____

QRS complex: _____

QT interval: _____

Other: _____

Interpretation: _____

3.

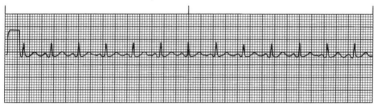

Atrial rhythm: _____

Ventricular rhythm: _____

Atrial rate: _____

Ventricular rate: _____

P wave: _____

PR interval: _____

QRS complex: _____

QT interval: _____

Other: _____

Interpretation: _____

4.

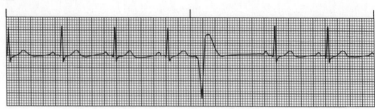

Atrial rhythm: _____

Ventricular rhythm: _____

Atrial rate: _____

Ventricular rate: _____

P wave: _____

PR interval: _____

QRS complex: _____

QT interval: _____

Other: _____

Interpretation: _____

5.

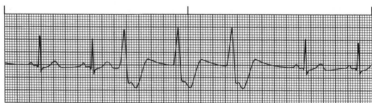

Atrial rhythm: _____

Ventricular rhythm: _____

Atrial rate: _____

Ventricular rate: _____

P wave: _____

PR interval: _____

QRS complex: _____

QT interval: _____

Other: _____

Interpretation: _____

6.

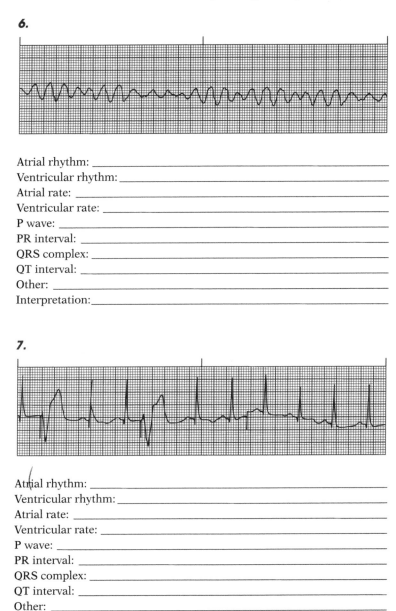

Atrial rhythm: _____

Ventricular rhythm: _____

Atrial rate: _____

Ventricular rate: _____

P wave: _____

PR interval: _____

QRS complex: _____

QT interval: _____

Other: _____

Interpretation: _____

7.

Atrial rhythm: _____

Ventricular rhythm: _____

Atrial rate: _____

Ventricular rate: _____

P wave: _____

PR interval: _____

QRS complex: _____

QT interval: _____

Other: _____

Interpretation: _____

8.

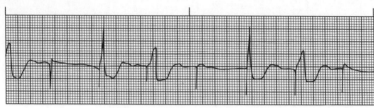

Atrial rhythm: _____

Ventricular rhythm: _____

Atrial rate: _____

Ventricular rate: _____

P wave: _____

PR interval: _____

QRS complex: _____

QT interval: _____

Other: _____

Interpretation:_____

9.

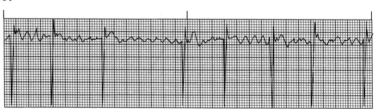

Atrial rhythm: _____

Ventricular rhythm: _____

Atrial rate: _____

Ventricular rate: _____

P wave: _____

PR interval: _____

QRS complex: _____

QT interval: _____

Other: _____

Interpretation:_____

10.

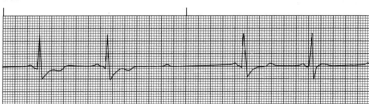

Atrial rhythm: _____

Ventricular rhythm: _____

Atrial rate: _____

Ventricular rate: _____

P wave: _____

PR interval: _____

QRS complex: _____

QT interval: _____

Other: _____

Interpretation: _____

11.

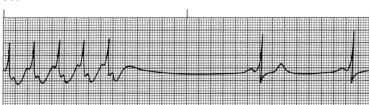

Atrial rhythm: _____

Ventricular rhythm: _____

Atrial rate: _____

Ventricular rate: _____

P wave: _____

PR interval: _____

QRS complex: _____

QT interval: _____

Other: _____

Interpretation: _____

12.

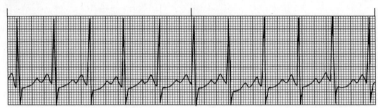

Atrial rhythm: _____

Ventricular rhythm: _____

Atrial rate: _____

Ventricular rate: _____

P wave: _____

PR interval: _____

QRS complex: _____

QT interval: _____

Other: _____

Interpretation: _____

13.

Atrial rhythm: _____

Ventricular rhythm: _____

Atrial rate: _____

Ventricular rate: _____

P wave: _____

PR interval: _____

QRS complex: _____

QT interval: _____

Other: _____

Interpretation: _____

14.

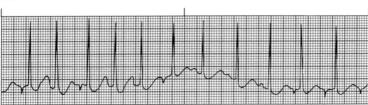

Atrial rhythm: _____

Ventricular rhythm: _____

Atrial rate: _____

Ventricular rate: _____

P wave: _____

PR interval: _____

QRS complex: _____

QT interval: _____

Other: _____

Interpretation: _____

15.

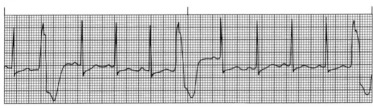

Atrial rhythm: _____

Ventricular rhythm: _____

Atrial rate: _____

Ventricular rate: _____

P wave: _____

PR interval: _____

QRS complex: _____

QT interval: _____

Other: _____

Interpretation: _____

16.

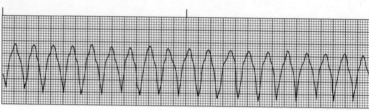

Atrial rhythm: _____

Ventricular rhythm: _____

Atrial rate: _____

Ventricular rate: _____

P wave: _____

PR interval: _____

QRS complex: _____

QT interval: _____

Other: _____

Interpretation: _____

17.

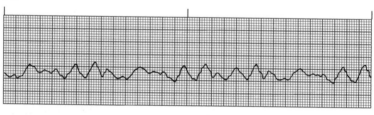

Atrial rhythm: _____

Ventricular rhythm: _____

Atrial rate: _____

Ventricular rate: _____

P wave: _____

PR interval: _____

QRS complex: _____

QT interval: _____

Other: _____

Interpretation: _____

18.

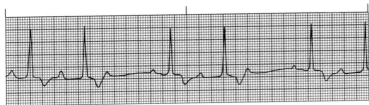

Atrial rhythm: _____

Ventricular rhythm: _____

Atrial rate: _____

Ventricular rate: _____

P wave: _____

PR interval: _____

QRS complex: _____

QT interval: _____

Other: _____

Interpretation: _____

19.

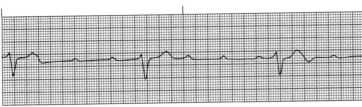

Atrial rhythm: _____

Ventricular rhythm: _____

Atrial rate: _____

Ventricular rate: _____

P wave: _____

PR interval: _____

QRS complex: _____

QT interval: _____

Other: _____

Interpretation: _____

20.

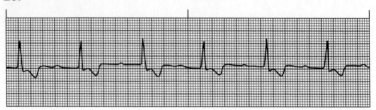

Atrial rhythm: _____

Ventricular rhythm: _____

Atrial rate: _____

Ventricular rate: _____

P wave: _____

PR interval: _____

QRS complex: _____

QT interval: _____

Other: _____

Interpretation: _____

■ Sharpening interpretation skills: Answers

1.

Atrial rhythm: Regular, except for missing PQRST complex

Ventricular rhythm: Regular, except for missing PQRST complex

Atrial rate: 50 beats/minute; underlying rate 60 beats/minute

Ventricular rate: 50 beats/minute

P wave: Normal size and configuration; absent during pause

PR interval: 0.20 second

QRS complex: 0.08 second

T wave: Normal configuration; absent during pause

QT interval: 0.40 second

Other: None

Interpretation: Sinus arrest

2.

Atrial rhythm: Irregular

Ventricular rhythm: Irregular

Atrial rate: 60 beats/minute; underlying rate 88 beats/minute

Ventricular rate: 90 beats/minute

P wave: None with premature ventricular contractions (PVCs); present with QRS complexes

PR interval: 0.16 second

QRS complex: Underlying rate 0.08 second; 0.16 second with PVCs

T wave: Normal configuration; opposite direction with PVCs

QT interval: 0.42 second
Other: None
Interpretation: Normal sinus rhythm with trigeminal PVCs

3.
Atrial rhythm: Regular
Ventricular rhythm: Regular
Atrial rate: 125 beats/minute
Ventricular rate: 125 beats/minute
P wave: Normal size and configuration
PR interval: 0.14 second
QRS complex: 0.08 second
T wave: Normal configuration
QT interval: 0.32 second
Other: None
Interpretation: Sinus tachycardia

4.
Atrial rhythm: Irregular
Ventricular rhythm: Irregular
Atrial rate: 60 beats/minute; underlying rate 71 beats/minute
Ventricular rate: 70 beats/minute
P wave: None with PVC; present with QRS complexes
PR interval: 0.16 second
QRS complex: 0.08 second; 0.14 second with PVC
T wave: Normal configuration
QT interval: 0.40 second
Other: None
Interpretation: Normal sinus rhythm with PVC

5.
Atrial rhythm: Irregular
Ventricular rhythm: Irregular
Atrial rate: 40 beats/minute; underlying rate 70 beats/minute
Ventricular rate: 70 beats/minute
P wave: None with PVCs; present with QRS complexes
PR interval: 0.16 second
QRS complex: 0.08 second; 0.16 second with PVCs
T wave: Normal configuration
QT interval: 0.40 second
Other: None
Interpretation: Normal sinus rhythm with run of PVCs

6.
Atrial rhythm: Absent
Ventricular rhythm: Chaotic
Atrial rate: Absent
Ventricular rate: Undetermined

P wave: Absent
PR interval: Unmeasurable
QRS complex: Indiscernible
T wave: Indiscernible
QT interval: Not applicable
Other: None
Interpretation: Ventricular fibrillation

7.

Atrial rhythm: Regular
Ventricular rhythm: Regular
Atrial rate: 90 beats/minute; underlying rate 107 beats/minute
Ventricular rate: 110 beats/minute
P wave: Present in normal QRS complexes
PR interval: 0.16 second
QRS complex: 0.08 second
T wave: Normal configuration
QT interval: 0.32 second
Other: Random pacemaker spikes
Interpretation: Sinus tachycardia with pacemaker failure to sense

8.

Atrial rhythm: Unmeasurable
Ventricular rhythm: Regular
Atrial rate: Unmeasurable
Ventricular rate: Paced rate 40 beats/minute; pacer fires at 75 beats/minute
P wave: Absent
PR interval: Unmeasurable
QRS complex: Unmeasurable
T wave: Unidentifiable
QT interval: Unmeasurable
Other: None
Interpretation: Paced rhythm with failure to capture

9.

Atrial rhythm: Irregular
Ventricular rhythm: Irregular
Atrial rate: Indiscernible
Ventricular rate: 60 beats/minute
P wave: Absent; fine fibrillation waves present
PR interval: Indiscernible
QRS complex: 0.08 second
T wave: Indiscernible
QT interval: Unmeasurable
Other: None
Interpretation: Atrial fibrillation

10.
Atrial rhythm: Regular
Ventricular rhythm: Irregular
Atrial rate: 50 beats/minute
Ventricular rate: 30 beats/minute
P wave: Normal; some not followed by QRS complexes
PR interval: 0.16 second and constant for conducted impulses
QRS complex: 0.08 second
T wave: Normal configuration; absent if QRS complexes are absent
QT interval: 0.40 second
Other: None
Interpretation: Type II second-degree atrioventricular (AV) block

11.
Atrial rhythm: Irregular
Ventricular rhythm: Irregular
Atrial rate: 60 beats/minute
Ventricular rate: 70 beats/minute
P wave: Rate and configuration varies
PR interval: Varies with rhythm
QRS complex: 0.10 second
T wave: Configuration varies
QT interval: Configuration varies
Other: None
Interpretation: Sick sinus syndrome

12.
Atrial rhythm: Regular
Ventricular rhythm: Regular
Atrial rate: 110 beats/minute
Ventricular rate: 110 beats/minute
P wave: Normal size and configuration
PR interval: 0.16 second
QRS complex: 0.10 second
T wave: Normal configuration
QT interval: 0.36 second
Other: None
Interpretation: Sinus tachycardia

13.
Atrial rhythm: Regular
Ventricular rhythm: Regular
Atrial rate: 270 beats/minute
Ventricular rate: 70 beats/minute
P wave: Saw-tooth edged
PR interval: Unmeasurable
QRS complex: 0.10 second
T wave: Unidentifiable

QT interval: Unidentifiable
Other: None
Interpretation: Atrial flutter (4:1 block)

14.
Atrial rhythm: Irregular
Ventricular rhythm: Irregular
Atrial rate: About 150 beats/minute
Ventricular rate: About 150 beats/minute
P wave: Size and configuration vary
PR interval: Rate varies
QRS complex: 0.08 second
T wave: Inverted
QT interval: 0.22 second
Other: None
Interpretation: Multifocal atrial tachycardia

15.
Atrial rhythm: Irregular
Ventricular rhythm: Irregular
Atrial rate: 105 beats/minute
Ventricular rate: 105 beats/minute
P wave: Normal size and configuration, except during premature beat
PR interval: 0.16 second; unmeasurable for premature beat
QRS complex: 0.06 second
T wave: Normal configuration
QT interval: 0.36 second
Other: None
Interpretation: Sinus tachycardia with PVCs

16.
Atrial rhythm: Unmeasurable
Ventricular rhythm: Regular
Atrial rate: Unmeasurable
Ventricular rate: 187 beats/minute
P wave: Absent
PR interval: Unmeasurable
QRS complex: 0.18 second; wide and bizarre
T wave: Opposite direction of QRS complex
QT interval: Unmeasurable
Other: None
Interpretation: Ventricular tachycardia (monomorphic)

17.
Atrial rhythm: Absent
Ventricular rhythm: Chaotic
Atrial rate: Absent
Ventricular rate: Unmeasurable

P wave: Absent
PR interval: Absent
QRS complex: Indiscernible
T wave: Indiscernible
QT interval: Absent
Other: None
Interpretation: Ventricular fibrillation

18.

Atrial rhythm: Regular
Ventricular rhythm: Irregular
Atrial rate: 75 beats/minute
Ventricular rate: 50 beats/minute
P wave: Normal size and configuration
PR interval: Lengthens with each cycle until dropped
QRS complex: 0.06 second
T wave: Normal configuration
QT interval: 0.38 second
Other: None
Interpretation: Type 1 (Mobitz I or Wenckebach) second-degree AV block

19.

Atrial rhythm: Regular
Ventricular rhythm: Regular
Atrial rate: 90 beats/minute
Ventricular rate: 30 beats/minute
P wave: Normal size and configuration, except when hidden within
T wave
PR interval: Rate varies
QRS complex: 0.16 second
T wave: Normal configuration
QT interval: 0.56 second
Other: None
Interpretation: Third-degree AV block

20.

Atrial rhythm: Regular
Ventricular rhythm: Regular
Atrial rate: 60 beats/minute
Ventricular rate: 60 beats/minute
P wave: Normal size and configuration
PR interval: 0.36 second
QRS complex: 0.08 second
T wave: Normal configuration
QT interval: 0.40 second
Other: None
Interpretation: Normal sinus rhythm with first-degree AV block

■ *ECG challenge: Differentiating rhythm strips*

Differentiating ECG rhythm strips can often be a tricky proposition, especially when waveform patterns appear strikingly similar. These pairs of rhythm strips are among the most challenging to interpret. Test your knowledge and skill by correctly identifying each rhythm strip; answers begin on page 244.

1.

Rhythm strip A

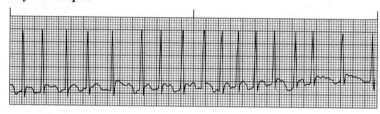

Rhythm strip A is: _____

Rhythm strip B

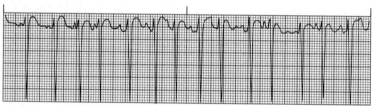

Rhythm strip B is: _____

2.
Rhythm strip A

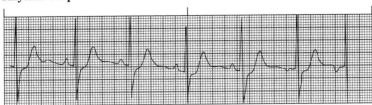

Rhythm strip A is: _____

Rhythm strip B

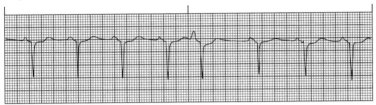

Rhythm strip B is: _____

3.
Rhythm strip A

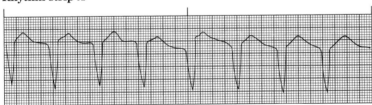

Rhythm strip A is: _____

Rhythm strip B

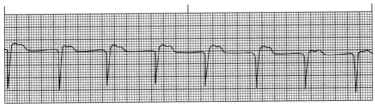

Rhythm strip B is: _____

4.

Rhythm strip A

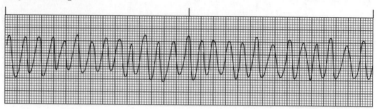

Rhythm strip A is: _____

Rhythm strip B

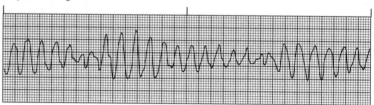

Rhythm strip B is: _____

5.

Rhythm strip A

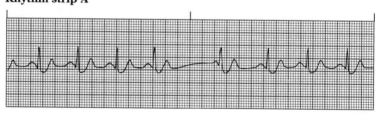

Rhythm strip A is: _____

Rhythm strip B

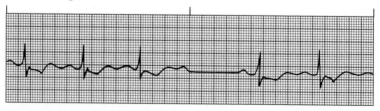

Rhythm strip B is: _____

6.

Rhythm strip A

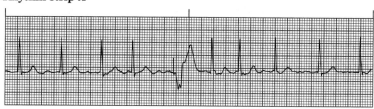

Rhythm strip A is: _____

Rhythm strip B

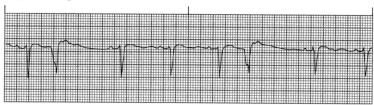

Rhythm strip B is: _____

■ *ECG challenge: Differentiating rhythm strips — Answers*

1.

Rhythm strip A: Atrial fibrillation
Rhythm strip B: Multifocal atrial tachycardia (MAT)

To help you decide whether a rhythm is atrial fibrillation, or the similar MAT, focus on the presence of P waves as well as the atrial and ventricular rhythms. You may find it helpful to look at a longer (greater than 6 seconds) rhythm strip.

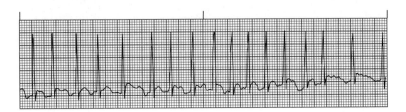

Atrial fibrillation

- Carefully look for discernible P waves before each QRS complex.
- If you can't clearly identify P waves, fibrillatory waves appear in place of P waves, and the rhythm is irregular, then the rhythm is probably atrial fibrillation.
- Carefully look at the rhythm, focusing on the R-R intervals. Remember that one of the hallmarks of atrial fibrillation is an irregularly irregular rhythm.

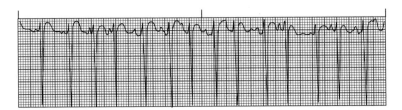

Multifocal atrial tachycardia

- P waves are present in MAT. Keep in mind, however, that the shape of the P waves will vary, with at least three different P wave shapes visible in a single rhythm strip.
- You should be able to see most, if not all, the various P wave shapes repeat.
- Although the atrial and ventricular rhythms are irregular, the irregularity generally isn't as pronounced as in atrial fibrillation.

2.

Rhythm strip A: Wandering pacemaker

Rhythm strip B: Premature atrial contraction (PAC)

Because PACs are commonly encountered, it's possible to mistake wandering pacemaker for PACs unless the rhythm strip is carefully examined. In such cases, you may find it helpful to look at a longer (greater than 6 seconds) rhythm strip.

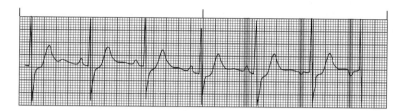

Wandering pacemaker

- Carefully examine the P waves. You must be able to identify at least three different shapes of P waves (see shaded areas above) in wandering pacemaker.
- Atrial rhythm varies slightly, with an irregular P-P interval. Ventricular rhythm also varies slightly, with an irregular R-R interval. These slight variations in rhythm result from the changing site of impulse formation.

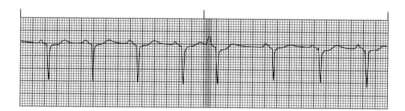

Premature atrial contraction

- The PAC occurs earlier than the sinus P wave, with an abnormal configuration when compared with a sinus P wave (see shaded area above). It's possible, but rare, to see multifocal PACs, which originate from multiple ectopic pacemaker sites in the atria. In this setting, the P waves have different shapes.
- With the exception of the irregular atrial and ventricular rhythms that result from the PAC, the underlying rhythm is usually regular.

3.

Rhythm strip A: Accelerated idioventricular rhythm
Rhythm strip B: Accelerated junctional rhythm

Accelerated idioventricular rhythm and accelerated junctional rhythm appear similar but have different causes. To distinguish between the two, closely examine the duration of the QRS complex and then look for P waves.

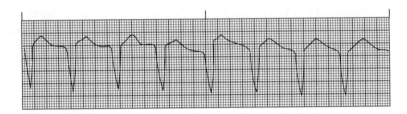

Accelerated idioventricular rhythm

■ The QRS duration will be greater than 0.12 second.
■ The QRS complex will have a wide and bizarre configuration.
■ P waves are usually absent.
■ The ventricular rate is generally between 40 and 100 beats/minute.

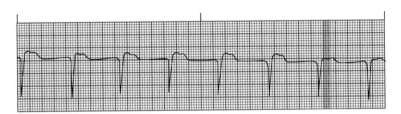

Accelerated junctional rhythm

■ The QRS duration and configuration are usually normal.
■ Inverted P waves generally occur before or after the QRS complex (see shaded area above). However, remember that P waves may also be buried within QRS complexes.
■ The ventricular rate is typically between 60 and 100 beats/minute.

4.

Rhythm strip A: Ventricular flutter
Rhythm strip B: Torsades de pointes

Torsades de pointes is a variant form of ventricular tachycardia, with a rapid ventricular rate that varies between 150 and 300 beats/minute. It's characterized by QRS complexes that gradually change back and forth, with the amplitude of each successive complex gradually increasing then decreasing. This results in an overall outline of the rhythm commonly described as *spindle-shaped.*

Ventricular flutter, although rarely recognized, results from the rapid, regular, repetitive beating of the ventricles. It's produced by a single ventricular focus firing at a rapid rate of 250 to 350 beats/minute. The hallmark of this arrhythmia is its smooth sine-wave appearance.

The illustrations shown here highlight key differences in the two arrhythmias.

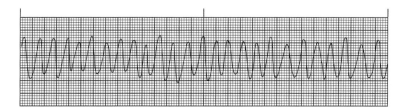

Ventricular flutter
■ Smooth sine-wave appearance

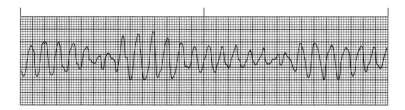

Torsades de pointes
■ Spindle-shaped appearance

5.

Rhythm strip A: Nonconducted PAC
Rhythm strip B: Type II second-degree AV block

An isolated P wave that doesn't conduct through to the ventricle (P wave without a QRS complex following it; see shaded areas in both illustrations below) may occur with either a nonconducted PAC or type II second-degree AV block. To differentiate the two, look for constancy of the P-P interval. Be aware that mistakenly identifying AV block as nonconducted PACs may have serious consequences. The latter is generally benign, whereas the former can be life-threatening.

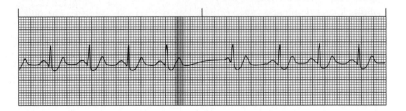

Nonconducted PAC

■ If the P-P interval, including the extra P wave, isn't constant, it's a nonconducted PAC.

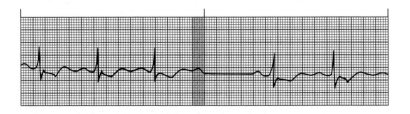

Type II second-degree AV block

■ If the P-P interval is constant, including the extra P wave, it's type II second-degree AV block.

6.

Rhythm strip A: Intermittent ventricular pacing
Rhythm strip B: Premature ventricular contraction

Knowing whether your patient has an artificial pacemaker will help you avoid mistaking a ventricular paced beat for a PVC. If your facility uses a monitoring system that eliminates artifact, make sure the monitor is set up correctly for a patient with a pacemaker. Otherwise, the pacemaker spikes may be eliminated as well.

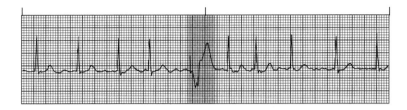

Intermittent ventricular pacing

- The paced ventricular complex will have a pacemaker spike preceding it (see shaded area above). You may need to look in different leads for a bipolar pacemaker spike because it's small and may be difficult to see.
- The paced ventricular complex of a properly functioning pacemaker won't occur early or prematurely. It will occur only when the patient's own ventricular rate falls below the rate set for the pacemaker.

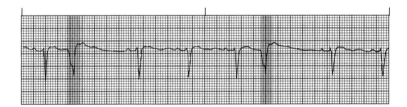

Premature ventricular contraction

- PVCs will occur prematurely and won't have pacemaker spikes preceding them (see shaded areas above).

Rapid reference to major arrhythmias

Sinus arrhythmia

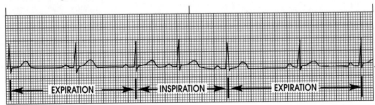

Features
- Rhythm irregular; varies with respiratory cycle
- P-P and R-R intervals shorter during inspiration, longer during expiration
- Normal P wave preceding each QRS complex

Sinus bradycardia

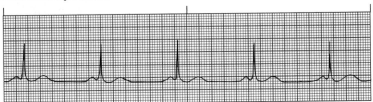

Features
- Rhythm regular
- Atrial and ventricular rates < 60 beats/minute
- Normal P wave preceding each QRS complex
- Normal QRS complex
- QT interval may be prolonged

Sinus tachycardia

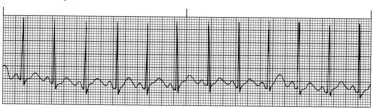

Features
- Rhythm regular
- Atrial and ventricular rates >100 beats/minute
- Normal P wave preceding each QRS complex
- Normal QRS complex
- QT interval commonly shortened

Sinus arrest

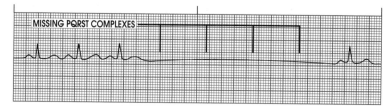

Features
- Rhythm normal, except for missing PQRST complexes
- P wave is periodically absent with entire PQRST complexes missing; when present, normal P wave precedes each QRS complex

Premature atrial contractions (PACs)

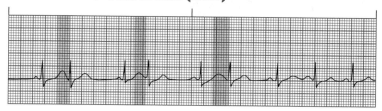

Features
- Premature, abnormal P waves (differ in configuration from normal P waves)
- QRS complexes after P waves, except in blocked PACs
- P wave often buried or identified in preceding T wave

Atrial tachycardia

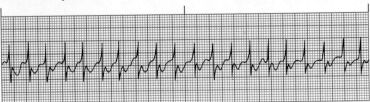

Features
- Rhythm regular if block is constant; irregular if not
- Rate 150 to 250 beats/minute
- P waves regular but hidden in preceding T wave; precede QRS complexes

Atrial flutter

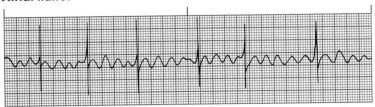

Features
- Atrial rhythm regular; ventricular rhythm variable
- Atrial rate 250 to 400 beats/minute; ventricular rate depends on degree of atrioventricular (AV) block
- Sawtooth P-wave configuration (flutter waves)

Atrial fibrillation

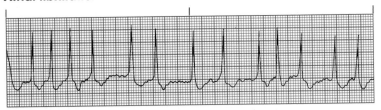

Features
- Atrial and ventricular rhythms grossly irregular
- Atrial rate > 400 beats/minute; ventricular rate varies
- No P waves; replaced by fine fibrillatory waves

Wandering pacemaker

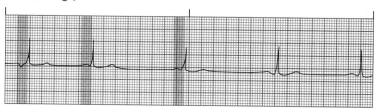

Features
- Rhythm irregular
- PR interval varies
- P waves change in configuration, indicating origin in sinoatrial node, atria, or AV junction (*Hallmark:* At least three different P wave configurations)

Premature junctional contractions (PJCs)

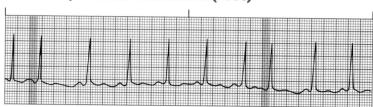

Features
- Rhythm irregular during PJCs
- P waves before, hidden in, or after QRS complexes; inverted if visible
- PR interval < 0.12 second, if P wave precedes QRS complex
- QRS configuration and duration normal

Junctional escape rhythm

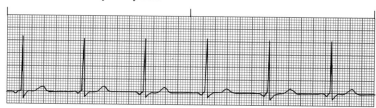

Features
- Rhythm regular
- Rate 40 to 60 beats/minute
- P waves before, hidden in, or after QRS complexes; inverted if visible
- PR interval < 0.12 second (measurable only if P wave appears before QRS complex)

Junctional tachycardia

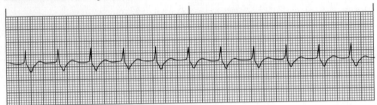

Features
- Rhythm regular
- Rate 100 to 200 beats/minute
- P waves before, hidden in, or after QRS complexes; inverted if visible

Premature ventricular contractions (PVCs)

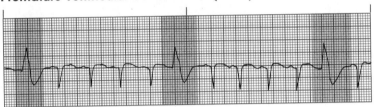

Features
- Underlying rhythm regular; P wave absent with PVCs
- Ventricular rhythm irregular during PVC
- QRS premature, usually followed by compensatory pause
- QRS complex wide and bizarre, duration > 0.12 second
- Premature QRS complexes occurring singly, in pairs, or in threes; possibly unifocal or multiformed
- Most ominous when clustered, multiformed, and with R wave on T pattern

Ventricular tachycardia

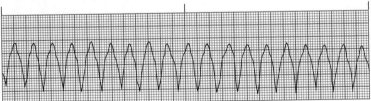

Features
- Atrial rhythm can't be determined; ventricular rhythm usually regular
- Ventricular rate 100 to 250 beats/minute
- QRS complexes wide and bizarre; duration > 0.12 second
- P waves indiscernible

Ventricular fibrillation

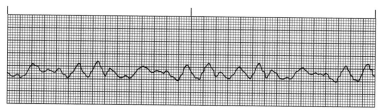

Features
- Atrial rhythm can't be determined
- Ventricular rhythm has no pattern, just chaotic fibrillatory waves
- Atrial and ventricular rates can't be determined
- No discernible P waves, QRS complexes, or T waves

Asystole

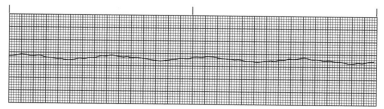

Features
- No atrial or ventricular rhythm or rate
- No discernible P waves, QRS complexes, or T waves

First-degree AV block

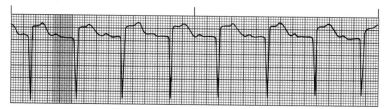

Features
- Rhythm regular
- PR interval > 0.20 second and constant
- P wave preceding each QRS complex; QRS complex normal

Type I second-degree AV block (Mobitz I, Wenckebach)

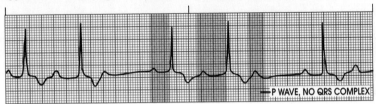

→ P WAVE, NO QRS COMPLEX

Features
- Atrial rhythm regular
- Ventricular rhythm irregular
- Atrial rate exceeds ventricular rate
- PR interval progressively longer with each cycle until a P wave appears without a QRS complex (dropped beat)

Type II second-degree AV block (Mobitz Type II)

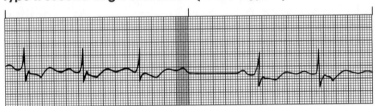

Features
- Atrial rhythm regular
- Ventricular rhythm possibly irregular, varying with degree of block
- P waves normal size and configuration; some not followed by QRS complex
- PR interval is constant for conducted beats
- QRS complexes periodically absent

Third-degree AV block (complete heart block)

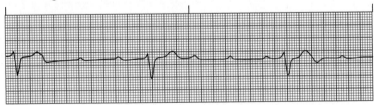

Features
- Atrial and ventricular rhythms regular
- Ventricular rate is 40 to 60 beats/minute (AV node origin); < 40 beats/minute (Purkinje system origin)
- No relationship between P waves and QRS complexes
- QRS complex normal (originating in AV node) or wide and bizarre (originating in Purkinje system)

Cardiac drug overview

Drug	Action	Indications	Adverse effects	Special considerations
adenosine (Adenocard)	■ Slows conduction through the atrioventricular (AV) node	Paroxysmal supraventricular tachycardia (PSVT)	■ Chest pain ■ Dyspnea ■ Flushing ■ Transient sinus bradycardia and ventricular ectopy	■ Monitor cardiac rate and rhythm. ■ A brief period of asystole (up to 15 seconds) may occur after rapid administration. ■ Rapidly follow each dose with a 20-ml saline flush. ■ Don't administer through a central line because a more prolonged asystole may result.
amiodarone (Cordarone)	■ Blocks sodium channels at rapid pacing frequencies and prolongs the duration and refractory period of the action potential	Life-threatening ventricular arrhythmias, such as recurrent ventricular fibrillation and recurrent, unstable ventricular tachycardia; may be used to control rate in supraventricular arrhythmias, particularly, atrial fibrillation, and atrial flutter	■ Bradycardia ■ Exacerbation of arrhythmia ■ Fever ■ Heart failure ■ Hepatotoxicity ■ Hyperthyroidism ■ Hypotension ■ Hypothyroidism ■ Nausea and vomiting ■ Ophthalmic abnormalities: Corneal microdeposits ■ Photosensitivity and skin discoloration ■ Pulmonary fibrosis	■ Closely monitor the patient during loading phase. ■ If the patient needs a dosage adjustment, monitor him for an extended time because of the drug's long and variable half-life and the difficulty in predicting the time needed to achieve new steady-state plasma drug level. ■ Administer oral doses with meals. ■ Monitor need to adjust dose of digoxin or warfarin. ■ Monitor pulmonary, liver, and thyroid function tests.

Drug	Action	Indications	Adverse effects	Special considerations
atropine	■ Blocks vagal effects on the sinoatrial (SA) and AV nodes and enhances conduction through the AV node and increases the heart rate	Symptomatic sinus bradycardia, AV block, asystole and bradycardic pulseless electrical activity (PEA)	■ Blurred vision ■ Dry mouth ■ Palpitations ■ Restlessness ■ Tachycardia ■ Urine retention	■ Monitor cardiac rate and rhythm. ■ Use with caution with myocardial ischemia. ■ Not recommended for third-degree AV block and infranodal type II second-degree AV block. ■ In adults, avoid doses less than 0.5 mg because of risk of paradoxical slowing. ■ Isn't effective in denervated transplanted hearts.
digoxin	■ Increases force and velocity of myocardial contraction; slows conduction through SA and AV nodes	Slows heart rate in sinus tachycardia from heart failure and controls rapid ventricular rate in patients with atrial fibrillation or flutter	■ AV block ■ Bradycardia ■ Headaches ■ Hypokalemia ■ Nausea and vomiting ■ Vision disturbances	■ Digoxin is extremely toxic, with a narrow margin of safety between therapeutic range and toxicity. ■ Vomiting is usually an early sign of drug toxicity. ■ Check apical pulse before giving drug and discontinue digoxin, as ordered, if patient's pulse rate falls below 60 beats/minute.
diltiazem (Cardizem)	■ Inhibits influx of calcium through the cell membrane, resulting in a depression of automaticity and conduction velocity in smooth and cardiac muscles ■ Different degrees of selectivity on vascular smooth muscle, myocardium, and conduction and pacemaker tissues	Atrial fibrillation, atrial flutter, atrial tachycardia	■ Abdominal discomfort ■ Acute hepatic injury ■ AV block ■ Bradycardia ■ Dizziness ■ Edema ■ Headache ■ Heart failure	■ Closely monitor the patient when starting therapy and during dosage adjustments. ■ Hypertensive patients treated with calcium channel blockers have a higher risk of heart attack than patients treated with diuretics or beta-adrenergic blockers. ■ Abrupt withdrawal may result in increased frequency and duration of chest pain.

Drug	Action	Indications	Adverse effects	Special considerations
diltiazem (continued)				■ Monitor cardiac and respiratory function. ■ Don't use for a patient with Wolff-Parkinson-White (WPW) syndrome or wide-QRS tachycardia of uncertain origin. ■ Concurrent I.V. administration with I.V. beta-adrenergic blocker may cause severe hypotension.
disopyramide (Norpace)	■ Decreases rate of diastolic depolarization and upstroke velocity; increases action potential duration; prolongs refractory period	Life-threatening ventricular arrhythmias such as sustained ventricular tachycardia	■ Chest pain ■ First-degree AV block ■ Hypotension ■ Long QT interval ■ Nausea ■ Widening of QRS complex	■ Monitor for arrhythmias and electrocardiogram (ECG) changes; notify physician of widened QRS complex or prolonged QT interval. ■ Disopyramide increases risk of death in patients with non–life-threatening ventricular arrhythmias. ■ Use cautiously in patients with WPW syndrome or bundle-branch block.
dofetilide (Tikosyn)	■ Blocks cardiac potassium channels; increases duration of action potential by delaying repolarization	Maintains sinus rhythm in patients with chronic atrial fibrillation or atrial flutter	■ Chest pain ■ Headache ■ Torsades de pointes	■ Don't use if baseline QTc is greater than 440 msec, if baseline heart rate is less than 50 beats/minute, or if severe renal impairment exists. ■ Must be initiated by cardiologist, with continuous ECG monitoring for at least 3 days. ■ Don't use with cimetidine, verapamil, ketoconazole, or trimethoprim.

Drug	Action	Indications	Adverse effects	Special considerations
epinephrine	■ Stimulates alpha and beta receptors in the sympathetic nervous system; relaxes bronchial smooth muscle by stimulating beta$_2$ receptors	Cardiac arrest (ventricular fibrillation (VF), pulseless ventricular tachycardia, asystole, PEA), symptomatic bradycardia, and for treatment of bronchospasm and anaphylaxis	■ Angina ■ Cerebral hemorrhage ■ Hypertension ■ Nervousness ■ Palpitations ■ Tachycardia	■ Monitor cardiac rate and rhythm and blood pressure because increased heart rate and blood pressure may cause myocardial ischemia. ■ Don't mix I.V. dose with alkaline solutions. ■ Give drug into a large vein to prevent irritation or extravasation at site.
flecainide (Tambocor)	■ Decreases excitability, conduction velocity and automaticity due to slowed atrial, AV node, His-Purkinje system, and intraventricular conduction	Ventricular arrhythmias, supraventricular arrhythmias (patients without coronary artery disease), and atrial fibrillation and atrial flutter	■ Dizziness ■ Dyspnea ■ Headache ■ Nausea ■ Ventricular arrhythmias (new or worsened) ■ Vision disturbances	■ Contraindicated in patients with impaired left-ventricular function. ■ Periodically monitor trough plasma levels because 40% is bound to plasma protein. ■ Increase dosage as ordered at intervals of more than 4 days in patients with renal disease. ■ Monitor for ECG changes, prolonged PR interval, widening QRS complex, and lengthening of QT interval.
ibutilide (Corvert)	■ Delays repolarization by activating slow, inward current (mostly sodium), which results in prolonged duration of atrial and ventricular action potential and refractoriness	Rapid conversion of recent-onset atrial fibrillation or atrial flutter	■ Headache ■ Hypotension ■ Nausea ■ Prolonged QT interval ■ Torsades de pointes ■ Worsening ventricular tachycardia	■ Stop drug infusion as ordered when arrhythmia stops, if ventricular tachycardia occurs, or if QT interval becomes markedly prolonged. ■ Perform continuous ECG monitoring for at least 4 hours after dose is completed because of proarrhythmic risk. ■ Check potassium and magnesium levels and correct before giving drug.

Drug	Action	Indications	Adverse effects	Special considerations
lidocaine (Xylocaine)	■ Shortens the refractory period and suppresses the automaticity of ectopic foci without affecting conduction of impulses through cardiac tissue	Acute ventricular arrhythmias, such as ventricular tachycardia and VF	■ Dizziness ■ Hallucinations ■ Nervousness ■ Seizures ■ Tachycardia ■ Tachypnea	■ Monitor cardiac rhythm and notify physician of prolonged PR interval and widened QRS complex. ■ Contraindicated in second- or third-degree AV block without pacing support, WPW syndrome, and Stokes-Adams syndrome. ■ Reduce drug dosage as ordered in patients with heart failure or liver disease. ■ Monitor patient closely for central nervous system changes.
moricizine (Ethmozine)	■ Shortens phase II and III repolarization, leading to decreased duration of the action potential and an effective refractory period	Life-threatening ventricular arrhythmias such as sustained ventricular tachycardia	■ Bradycardia ■ Dizziness ■ Headache ■ Nausea ■ Sustained ventricular tachycardia	■ Use cautiously in patients with sick sinus syndrome because of the possibility of sinus arrest. ■ The patient should be hospitalized for initial dosing and monitored for heart failure. ■ Give before meals because food delays rate of absorption.
procainamide (Procanbid, Pronestyl)	■ Produces a direct cardiac effect to prolong the refractory period of the atria and (to a lesser extent) the His-Purkinje system and the ventricles	Potentially life-threatening ventricular arrhythmias; and atrial fibrillation with rapid rate in WPW syndrome	■ Agranulocytosis ■ Diarrhea ■ Dizziness ■ Heart block ■ Hypotension ■ Liver failure ■ Lupus erythematosus-like syndrome ■ Nausea and vomiting	■ Monitor for arrhythmias and notify physician of widened QRS complex or prolonged QT interval. ■ Procainamide increases risk of death in patients with non–life-threatening arrhythmias. ■ Use with caution in patients with liver or kidney dysfunction. ■ Tell patient not to crush or break extended-release tablets.

Drug	Action	Indications	Adverse effects	Special considerations
propafenone (Rythmol)	■ Reduces up-stroke velocity of monophasic action potential ■ Reduces fast, inward current carried by sodium ions in Purkinje fibers ■ Increases diastolic excitability threshold ■ Prolongs effective refractory period	Life-threatening ventricular arrhythmias such as ventricular tachycardia when benefits of treatment outweigh risks	■ AV block ■ Constipation ■ Dizziness ■ Headache ■ Nausea and vomiting ■ Unusual taste ■ Ventricular tachycardia	■ Monitor liver and renal function studies. ■ Report significant widening of QRS complex and evidence of second- or third-degree AV block. ■ Increase dosage more gradually, as ordered, in elderly patients and patients with previous myocardial damage.
propranolol (Inderal)	■ Antiarrhythmic action results from beta-adrenergic receptor blockade as well as a direct membrane stabilization action on cardiac cells	Ventricular tachycardias, supraventricular arrhythmias, and premature ventricular contractions	■ AV block ■ Bradycardia ■ Heart failure ■ Hypotension ■ Light-headedness ■ Nausea and vomiting	■ Propranolol is also used for treatment of hypertension, angina pectoris, and myocardial infarction (MI). ■ Dosages may differ for hypertension, angina, or MI. ■ Check apical pulse before giving drug. If extremes in pulse rate occur, stop drug and notify physician immediately. ■ Report significant lengthening of PR interval and monitor for AV block. ■ Drug masks common signs and symptoms of shock and hypoglycemia. ■ Use cautiously in patients with reactive airway disease (asthma).

Drug	Action	Indications	Adverse effects	Special considerations
sotalol (Betapace)	■ Antiarrhythmic with beta-blocking effects and prolongation of the action potential ■ Slows AV nodal conduction and increases AV nodal refractoriness	Life-threatening ventricular arrhythmias; maintains sinus rhythm in patients with history of symptomatic atrial fibrillation or atrial flutter	■ Bradycardia ■ Chest pain ■ Dizziness ■ Fatigue ■ Palpitations ■ QT prolongation	■ Contraindicated in patients with bronchial asthma, sinus bradycardia, or second- or third-degree AV block without a pacemaker. ■ Perform ECG monitoring for at least 3 days when therapy starts. ■ Adjust dosage in renally impaired patients. ■ Monitor patient for QTc prolongation. ■ Administer drug when patient has an empty stomach.
vasopressin	■ Antidiuretic hormone acts at the cyclic adenosine monophosphate (cAMP) and increases permeability of renal tubular epithelium to water; at high doses, is a powerful vasoconstrictor of capillaries and small arterioles and may help maintain coronary perfusion pressure	Cardiac arrest with VF as an alternative to epinephrine	■ Bronchoconstriction ■ Chest pain ■ Hypersensitivity ■ Myocardial ischemia ■ Water intoxication	■ Monitor cardiac rhythm and blood pressure. ■ Assess for hypersensitivity reactions, including urticaria, angioedema, bronchoconstriction and anaphylaxis.

Selected references

Albert, N.M. "Cardiac Resynchronization Therapy through Biventricular Pacing in Patients with Heart Failure and Ventricular Dyssynchrony," *Critical Care Nurse* 23(3 Suppl):2-13, June 2003.

ECG Cards, 4th ed. Philadelphia: Lippincott Williams & Wilkins, 2005.

ECG Interpretation: An Incredibly Easy Pocket Guide. Philadelphia: Lippincott Williams & Wilkins, 2006.

Fuster, V., et al. (Eds). *Atherothrombosis and Coronary Artery Disease,* 2nd ed. Philadelphia: Lippincott Williams & Wilkins, 2005.

Geiter, Jr., H.B. "Understanding Wolff-Parkinson-White and Preexcitation Syndromes," *Nursing* 33(11):32cc1-32cc4, November 2003.

Hazinski, M.F., et al. (Eds). *Handbook of Emergency Cardiovascular Care for Healthcare Providers.* Dallas: American Heart Association, 2004.

Hesselson, A. *Simplified Interpretation of Pacemaker ECGs.* Elmsford, N.Y.: Blackwell/Futura, 2003.

Khan, M.G. *Rapid ECG Interpretation,* 2nd ed. Philadelphia: W.B. Saunders Co., 2003.

LeRoy, S.S. "Long QT Syndrome and Other Repolarization-related Dysrhythmias," *AACN Clinical Issues Advanced Practice in Acute and Critical Care: Electrophysiology and Device Therapy* 15(3): 419-31, July-September 2004.

Mair, M. "Emergency: Monophasic and Biphasic Defibrillators," *AJN* 103(8):58-60, August 2003.

Mastering ACLS, 2nd ed. Philadelphia: Lippincott Williams & Wilkins, 2006.

Morton, S., et al. *Critical Care Nursing: A Holistic Approach,* 8th ed. Philadelphia: Lippincott Williams & Wilkins, 2005.

Nursing2006 Drug Handbook, 26th ed. Philadelphia: Lippincott Williams & Wilkins, 2006.

Pyne, C.C. "Classification of Acute Coronary Syndromes Using the 12-lead Electrocardiogram as a Guide," *AACN Clinical Issues Advanced Practice in Acute and Critical Care: Advanced Assessment* 15(4):558-67, October-December 2004.

Rakel, R.E., and Bope, E.T. *Conn's Current Therapy 2005.* Philadelphia: W.B. Saunders Co., 2005.

Shea, J.B. "Quality of Life Issues in Patients with Implantable Cardioverter Defibrillators Driving, Occupation and Recreation," *AACN Clinical Issues Advanced Practice in Acute and Critical Care: Electrophysiology and Device Therapy* 15(3):478-89, July-September 2004.

Tierney, L.M., et al. *Current Medical Diagnosis and Treatment,* 44th ed. New York: McGraw-Hill/Appleton & Lange, 2005.

Woods, S.L., et al. *Cardiac Nursing,* 5th ed. Philadelphia: Lippincott Williams & Wilkins, 2005.

Index

A

AAI pacemaker, 196-197, 196i
Accelerated idioventricular
    rhythm, 79-80, 81, 81i
  distinguishing, from accelerat-
      ed junctional rhythm, 82i
Accelerated junctional rhythm,
    73, 74i
  distinguishing, from acceler-
      ated idioventricular
      rhythm, 82i
AC interference as monitor
    problem, 43, 45t
Action potential curves, 13, 14i
  antiarrhythmic drugs and, 182,
      183i, **C4**
Acute coronary syndromes,
    118-135
  causes of, 118
  ECG characteristics of,
      120-121, 121i, 122-124i,
      123-124, 126
  interventions for, 126, 128-129
  pathophysiology of, 118, 119i
  risk factors for, 118-119
  signs and symptoms of, 120
Adenosine, 259t
Adult, position of heart in, 2
AFib. *See* Atrial fibrillation.
Afterdepolarization, 17, 46, 157
Afterload, 11i, 12
Amiodarone, 259t

Angina. *See also* Acute coronary
    syndromes *and* Wellens
    syndrome.
  ECG characteristics of,
      120-121, 121i
  forms of, 120
  signs and symptoms of, 120
  vessel occlusion in, 118
Anterior hemiblock, 143-145,
    143i, 144i
Anterior wall myocardial infarc-
    tion, 130, 131i
Antiarrhythmics, 182-190
  action potential and, 182,
      183i, **C4**
  class I, 184-186, 185i, 186i, 187i
  class II, 186-178, 188i
  class III, 188, 189i
  class IV, 189, 190i
  classifying, 182
  distribution and clearance
      of, 183
  proarrhythmic effects of,
      183-184
Antitachycardia pacing, 214t
Aortic valve, 5i, 6
Arrhythmias
  nonpharmacologic treatment
      for, 192-221
  pharmacologic treatment for,
      182-191
  versus dysrhythmia, 33

---

t refers to a table; i refers to an illustration; **boldface** refers to a full-color page.

t refers to a table; i refers to an illustration; **boldface** refers to a full-color page.

C

Calcium channel blockers. *See*
Class IV antiarrhythmics.
Calcium imbalance. *See*
Hypercalcemia *and*
Hypocalcemia.
Caliper method of measuring
rhythm, 35i
Cardiac cells
depolarization-repolarization
cycle and, 12-15, 13i, 14i
key characteristics of, 12
Cardiac conduction system,
15-17, 16i
abnormal impulse conduction
and, 17
Cardiac cycle, 9-11
diastole in, 9-11, 10i
phases of, 10i
systole in, 10i, 11
Cardiac drugs, 182-191, 259-265t
Cardiac enzymes and proteins,
release of, in myocardial
infarction, 128i
Cardiac output, 11-12
in elderly person, 3
Cardiac resynchronization therapy. *See* Biventricular pacing.
Cardiac veins, 8i, 9
Cardiovascular system
anatomy of, 2-9, 3i, 4i, 5i, 8i
physiology of, 9-17, 10i, 11i,
13i, 14i, 16i
Cardioversion, 214t
Carotid sinus massage as paroxysmal atrial tachycardia
intervention, 62
Chaotic atrial rhythm. *See* Multifocal atrial tachycardia.
Chest leads, 100
normal findings in, 110-111i
views of the heart monitored
by, 100i
Chest pain
in angina, 120
in myocardial infarction, 120

Child, position of heart in, 2-3
Chordae tendineae, 5i, 6
Circulation
collateral, 8-9
pulmonic, 6-7
systemic, 7
Circumflex artery, 7-8, 8i
Class I antiarrhythmics, 184-187
action potential and, **C4**
Class IA antiarrhythmics, 184
ECG effects of, 184-185, 185i
Class IB antiarrhythmics, 185
ECG effects of, 185, 186i
Class IC antiarrhythmics, 186
ECG effects of, 186, 187i
Class II antiarrhythmics, 186-187
action potential and, **C4**
ECG effects of, 187, 188i
Class III antiarrhythmics, 188
action potential and, **C4**
ECG effects of, 188, 189i
Class IV antiarrhythmics, 189
action potential and, **C4**
ECG effects of, 189, 190i
Coding system for pacemak-
ers, 195
Collateral circulation, 8-9
Complete heart block, 95-96,
96i, 258i
Conductivity, cardiac cells
and, 12
Contractility, cardiac cells
and, 12
Coronary arteries, 7-9, 8i
Coronary blood supply, 7-9, 8i
Coronary sinus, 8i, 9
Countdown method for calculat-
ing heart rate, 37t

D

DDD pacemaker, 198i, 199
Defibrillation, 214t
Defibrillators, types of, **C1**
Degree method for determining
electrical axis, 114, 116i
Delayed afterdepolarization,
17, 157

---

t refers to a table; i refers to an illustration; **boldface** refers to a full-color page.

t refers to a table; i refers to an illustration; **boldface** refers to a full-color page.

---

t refers to a table; i refers to an illustration; **boldface** refers to a full-color page.

---

t refers to a table; i refers to an illustration; **boldface** refers to a full-color page.

t refers to a table; i refers to an illustration; **boldface** refers to a full-color page.

---

t refers to a table; i refers to an illustration; **boldface** refers to a full-color page.

t refers to a table; i refers to an illustration; **boldface** refers to a full-color page.